COUNTING FOR SOMETHING IN MENTAL HEALTH SERVICES

Counting for Something in Mental Health Services

Effective user feedback

Edited by

ROB LEIPER
VIDA FIELD

Avebury

Aldershot · Brookfield USA · Hong Kong · Singapore · Sydney

Published by
Avebury
Ashgate Publishing Limited
Gower House
Croft Road
Aldershot
Hants GU11 3HR
England

Ashgate Publishing Company
Old Post Road
Brookfield
Vermont 05036
USA

British Library Cataloguing in Publication Data

Counting for Something in Mental Health Services:
Effective User Feedback
    I. Leiper, Rob II. Field, Vida
    362.2

ISBN 1 85628 477 8

Printed and Bound in Great Britain by
Athenaeum Press Ltd, Newcastle upon Tyne.

Contents

List of contributors

Ingrid Barker: is a Consultant with the Centre for Mental Heath Services Development and Mental Health Services Manager for Croydon. She is a qualified social worker with substantial experience in the voluntary sector, particulary in establishing self-advocacy projects. More recently she has been working as a manager in the NHS and has been a purchaser of community care services.

Marion Beeforth: is a long-term user of Mental Health services and is a former chair of the Brighton INSIGHT independent user group. She has been very active in user participation work for some years.

Edna Conlan: is a member of the Milton Keynes Advocacy Group and Chairperson of the United Kingdom Advocacy Network. She has worked as a lecturer, trainer and researcher for the Open University and the London School of Economics and is a consultant for the Centre of Mental Health Services Development at King's College.

Vida Field: is Policy and Information Manager at Research and Development for Psychology (RDP).

Richard Grover: is a freelance consultant and researcher specializing in community care issues. He was previously Director of the Peter Bedford Trust.

Victoria Heckels: is Project Coordinator with CASPE Research. She has developed patient satisfaction systems for acute psychiatric inpatients and for accident and emergency patients and is currently developing a patient satisfaction system for use in the three Special Hospitals.

Dr Frank Holloway: is Consultant Psychiatrist, Maudsley Hospital and St Giles' Day Hospital. His research and clinical interests focus on services for people with severe long-term mental illnesses. He was involved in a successfully completed hospital closure programme and is now developing a Model Case Management Service.

Lyn Jones: is Director of Scottish Health Feedback, an independent organization which specializes in gathering the views of patients and other health service users. SHF works for Health Boards, Units, and Health Councils all over Scotland, covering all forms of primary, community and acute care as well as mental health services.

Leonie Kellaher: is Senior Research Officer/Senior Lecturer at the University of North London and is Director of the Centre for Environmental and Social Studies (CESSA) there.

Alison Kerruish: is a Research Fellow, Centre for the Applied Psychology of Social Care and Project Manger for the Quality for People Project, has worked in NHS Quality Assurance related research for seven years. Her main interest is in the development of services through research carried out in conjunction with service users.

Rob Leiper: is Deputy Director of the S. E. Thames Regional Clinical Psychology Course and the former project director for quality assurance at RDP.

Steve Pilling: is a Clinical Psychologist at the Whittington Hospital, London.

James Raftery: is a Health Economist in the Department of Clinical Epidemiology at St Georges Hospital, London.

Shulamit Ramon, PhD: is Course Director for the course 'Mental Health Work with the Continued Care Client', at the London School of Economics and is a Senior Lecturer in Social Work, LSE and researcher in community care.

Sally Robbins: is a Clinical Psychologist who specializes in working with elderly people. She has recently become Elderly Services Manager for Priority Care Services in Maidstone and is actively involved in developing user feedback within the service.

Liz Sayce: is Policy Director of MIND, the National Association for Mental Health. MIND works throughout England and Wales to promote mental health and to improve the quality of life of people with mental health problems. Liz Sayce has a background in social work and mental health research and has published work on a number of issues in British mental health policy, including community mental health centres, psychiatric case registers and user involvement.

Helen Smith: is Senior Lecturer, Centre for the Applied Psychology of Social Care. She has substantial experience of service development for people with long-term mental health problems and has a particular interest in user involvement and quality assurance.

Dr David Somekh: is Clinical Director for Mental Health, Ravensbourne NHS Trust, Bromley.

Maggie Veitch: worked as Research Officer on the development of IQA after moving to CESSA (University of North London) from a Senior Practitioner's post in an inner London Social Service Department, and has recently returned to development work with children in Scotland.

Yvonne Webb: is Senior Research Manager for the *FACE* project based at the Research Unit, Royal College of Psychiatrists.

Foreword

There are growing expectations from an increasingly vociferous public that human care services will take into account the views of users in the way services are planned, organized and delivered. Mental health services in particular have not traditionally taken the opinions of service recipients very seriously. A dismissive attitude stems, in part, from the long recognized association of mental health problems with poverty and other social ills which places mentally disordered people at the bottom of the social hierarchy, unable to influence the things done to them by statutory agencies, and in part from more fundamental attitudinal problems to the stigma of mental disorder.

There remains in many in-patient units and mental health centres in Britain an attitude that only professionals know what is in the 'best interests' of the 'patients'. The attitude problem is compounded by the fact that 12 per cent or so of in-patients are admitted for assessment or treatment against their wishes, under the provisions of the Mental Health Act. It is important to be explicit about when users' views are to be set aside in the interests of their future health or safety, and important also to realize that 'sectioned' patients, or those with a degree of mental incapacity, still have opinions which should be heard and taken into account.

A further confounding issue is that users of the services and their relatives do not always agree on what services should be provided or how an individual's future should be planned. The relatives of users, whose own lives may be significantly changed as a result of supporting their mentally ill relatives, have a right to be consulted and to contribute to the process of professional care planning, but generally the users' views must be given priority. Services must recognize and manage this tension between users and families.

Service users must make a contribution to planning their own care and can also, through surveys of groups of users, feed in their own experiences of the care they receive to the wider quality assurance process. If the right management mechanisms are in place, users' surveys can become an essential part of the planning process. Few authorities have yet moved far in this direction, but as new purchasing authorities flex their muscles of independence from local providers and seek ways of enhancing the quality content of contract specifications, it will be increasingly important to approach the problem of tapping user opinion by a methodologically sound process. It is crucial to use rigorous research methods to assess users' views if valid information is to be gained. The influence of one or two vociferous, but atypical, users on consultation exercises can seriously skew the findings of poorly designed surveys.

The experiences of the authors of this book provide excellent examples of a range of approaches that have already proved interesting, and in many cases sufficiently successful to encourage the participating organization to greater user involvement. This practical introduction to the topic will be of value to clinicians, managers and service planners in both statutory and independent sector agencies.

Professor Elaine Murphy
United Medical and Dental Schools
Guy's Hospital

Acknowledgements

Many of the contributions to this book were originally presented at a conference held by RDP (Research and Development for Psychiatry), and we would like to thank the participants for their contributions on the day which informed rewriting and editing of the papers. RDP is an independent research organization which aims to improve the quality of care for people with long-term mental health problems by the evaluation of service developments and the dissemination of the results of that research. We appreciate the help of RDP staff in the typing and correction of the manuscripts. Particular credit is due to Maureen McManus for the preparation of the camera ready copy.

Rob Leiper and Vida Field

Introduction: Listening to the voices of experience

Vida Field and Rob Leiper

Interest in ways of involving the 'consumer' in all areas of the public services has increased to an extraordinary extent in recent years. This represents a significant shift in the climate within which those services exist and it constitutes a considerable pressure for change in the internal culture of all our public institutions. This is a change which has become a 'movement', a movement with two quite different strands to it. On the one hand, there is a move from the top down to make services consumer oriented. It is represented particularly in the wave of published Charters, specifying the rights of consumers to certain standards of service and providing clearer procedures for making complaints. It adopts the language of 'customer focus' and takes a 'technological' approach by employing an array of systematic methodologies of quality assurance to guarantee standards and to feed back the views of people who have received a service. Such is the wave of interest in these techniques that consumer orientation has become a fashion, the latest buzz, and such is the pressure to undertake initiatives related to these expectations that it becomes increasingly difficult to distinguish modishness, compliance and public relations from a real concern with being responsive to the needs of service users.

At the same time, another strand of this culture change has come from the bottom up. This is an array of initiatives which might be grouped together as the users movement. Increasingly users have been making common cause with each other and asserting their right to be heard and to be involved in the planning of their care and the operation of the services they receive. Advocacy on an individual basis has developed in tandem with a collective movement to redress power imbalances and to change the shape and content of mental health services. The most common manifestations have been patients' councils, user forums and advocacy groups, examples of which are now to be found in many different parts of the country, following the pioneering work in Nottingham,

1

Brighton and Milton Keynes (Barker & Peck, 1988). Three national co-ordinating networks have been set up to provide a louder voice for users' views on their treatment and the services on offer and to encourage the development of local user organizations. Whilst none of these organizations would claim to 'represent' all users and they would differ in the extent to which they are prepared to work within the system, there is agreement that users should have greater control over their lives and the right to influence both individual treatment and the pattern of services.

The coming together of these different pressures for change has generated a demand within the mental health services for guidance on 'how to do it' – often a wish for ready-made tools, techniques and systems by which to obtain input from service users. Although several different approaches to involving consumers are outlined here, this book is not that manual of methods. A recent volume by McIver (1991) for the King's Fund Centre does provide considerable guidance of that kind and it suggests a variety of approaches by which the views of mental health service users might be obtained and utilized. Our intention in this volume is broader than that. It is to present differing points of view and to generate dialogue and debate about the place of 'consumer feedback' in mental health services, about the value and limitations of the various approaches that might be taken to it, and about the assumptions and goals behind the rhetoric with which these approaches are presented. We do not pretend to provide a conclusion to this debate, only the opportunity to learn from a diversity of experience and points of view.

This is an unapologetically diverse collection of papers. It is written in different voices and with different styles; it includes the sceptical and the empirically grounded through the pragmatic to the passionate and visionary; it covers a wide range of institutional positions and of perspectives spanning the users of services, professional practitioners, managers, service purchasers, researchers and organizational consultants. This diversity of perspective not only reflects the very widespread interest in these issues throughout the services, but it also provides a route into understanding some of the complexities and indeed the conflicts inherent in this area. What unites all the contributors is a commitment to improving mental health services and a respectful attention to the experiences of the people who use them.

However, this commitment means that the diversity of contributors does not quite cover the full range of points of view. Some members of the users movement cannot bring themselves to believe that the conventional public services can be fundamentally improved. They feel that current mental health provision is based on an inappropriate medical perspective which inevitably leads to an unhelpful view of their distress and interventions based on this 'illness model' compound that distress. They see current services as inherently oppressive and abusive in spite of any expressed good intentions and believe that only alternative services run by users can avoid being so. Consequently contributing to a book such as this would have no validity for those in the users movement who see things in this light. Their voice must, as it were, be heard only by its absence.

The diversity within the book is nevertheless very real and contains within it an array of differences in core values and focal concerns which may at times be bewildering. Nonetheless, a number of underlying themes and issues recur throughout many of the papers, whilst the way different authors relate to them depends on their reasons for seeking feedback and on the ways they are involved in the mental health system. As an introduction to thinking about these divergent points of view and an aid to keeping in mind some core issues, we will briefly outline those which strike us as central.

The issue which most immediately and commonly commands attention is that of method, the search for techniques by which to obtain user input, the 'how to do it' question. On the one hand this is a commendable desire to learn from the hard won experience of other people. It is perhaps also a wish to 'get it right'. Never far from the surface, however, is a sense of apprehension underlying this question. We feel that it may be helpful to start by acknowledging some of this and by suggesting that the reader may wish to keep an eye open for some of its sources. There is a good deal of confusion due to the extent and speed of the institutional changes facing services. Some clear pathways through would provide relief from this uncertainty. Perhaps services also posess a sense of collective guilt that they have failed their users in significant ways in the past by not listening to their experience. Users may appear as a threat and be seen as accusers of real or imagined sins. That sense of threat is further exaggerated by the extent that people labelled as mentally ill have in the past (and now) carried frightening aspects of society's own concerns – that is have been used as scapegoats. In these circumstances real dialogue with users is unconsciously a potentially frightening experience. Technique, with the sense of distance, certainty and authority that it can confer, is likely to be a convenient defence in the face of such anxiety.

Nevertheless, there are important technical considerations about how best to make services more responsive. There is however a danger of polarizing the debate about method, arguably in response to these very anxieties. On the one hand, methods of 'consumer feedback' tend to emphazise the accurate assessment of representative user views and so put a premium on methodologies for collecting them. Such approaches tend to de-emphasize the detail of structures for responding to these views and acting upon them. They pay little attention to the issue of the complex relationships inherent in making these changes. This is the starting point for the opposite pole in the debate about technique, which emphasizes 'user involvement'. In this, concern is directed towards the structures by which the planning and the day-to-day operation of services are undertaken, and ways are sought by which users may be organized and represented so as to influence decisions. James Raftery (Chapter 12) and Ingrid Barker (Chapter 13) emphasize these differing concerns in relation to the process of commissioning services. Both approaches, however, face substantial problems of implementation in practice. Yvonne Webb (Chapter 2) points out the many methodological challenges faced by feedback methodologies, while Marion Beeforth (Chapter 10) discusses the numerous personal and practical difficulties faced in truly attempting to influence services through user involvement.

In fact all serious approaches to obtaining input from the service user are faced with these issues of method and structure and of combining them effectively. Information must be obtained which is relevant and accurate while changes at various levels in the service must be pursued through committed action. This is the essence of constructive quality assurance processes and in Chapters 3 to 7 a variety of authors (Heckels, Jones, Pilling, Kellaher and Veitch, Kerruish and Smith) give accounts of the experience of adopting different approaches to this task. The relatively paucity of careful and objective evaluations of the success of quality assurance programmes is striking. They are too often presented in an idealized way in which good intentions and high hopes are prominent. We have sought reasonably frank and self-critical accounts of quality assurance programmes which reflect the real learning available from the experience of attempting constructively to obtain user input.

Such experience 'on the ground' inevitably leads to an understanding of the substantial difficulties which lie in the path of change. This is another theme underlying many of the contributions. In part this reflects the inevitable difficulties of influencing and promoting organizational change and development. This is the keynote of Leiper's concluding chapter and of Somekh's (Chapter 16) account of contrasting programmes in different districts. The increased expectation of user input is itself an enormous change and the new contracting arrangements within mental health services are, from the commissioner's point of view, extraordinary opportunities to exert a beneficial influence on service provision, as both Barker and Raftery point out. However, Somekh and Leiper both draw attention to the simultaneous difficulties that rapid organizational change, imposed from without, creates for planned change within service organizations. Understandably, many of the calls for change in mental health services come from outside. A danger of this can be that the sheer difficulty of work with people in extreme states of distress may be overlooked. These difficulties which staff face in isolated and under-resourced situations underlie many of the institutional practices and the

4

abuses which seem so obviously unsatisfactory from the outside. Understanding these practices as adaptations to the pressures of the work makes their rigidity more comprehensible and explains why many institutions are so intractable to change programmes. User input to services will only create sustainable change when such internal difficulties are understood and dealt with.

Consideration of change and influence inevitably raises the issue of power, too seldom explicitly discussed in relation to quality assurance programmes. Richard Grover (Chapter 8) points out how exploitive power relationships underlie many of the polarized and inflexible practices within mental health and other welfare services, and construes the role of quality assurance as essentially one of mediation which can break down such rigid distinctions. The call for user empowerment is thus a call for mutual respect and negotiation. However, some differences in power and some very real conflicts of interest do exist within the public services and are ignored at our peril. The call for user-run services is made in the hope of circumventing these inevitable differentials and conflicts, but arguably differences of interest and issues of authority would persist: some users would be more equal than others. This is to say that within the mental health services generally there are conflicts between the interests of different stakeholders which are not readily resolvable but which can only be negotiated to achieve some currently acceptable balance.

Many of these differences of interest are entirely honourable and represent the various perspectives of differing responsibilities within the system. Thus an underlying issue is the sheer complexity of issues of mental health treatment, perhaps even more than in other areas of the public health services. Hence, some authors from professional backgrounds but with roles which endeavour to improve common practice such as Shula Ramon (Chapter 15), emphasize the experiences of service users and both the civil rights of patients and their human right to respect; whereas other practioners such as Frank Holloway (Chapter 9) and Sally Robbins (Chapter 11), though respectful, alert us to the difficult realities and tensions that professional practice faces them with. Some workers such as Liz Sayce (Chapter 14) have it as a major role to promote ideals and policies on which to found a better service, whereas those writers concerned with quality assurance systems are more oriented to the possibilities and difficulties of producing pragmatic change in individual service settings. Perhaps particularly difficult to encompass is the underlying tension between understanding and supporting the experience and needs of individual sufferers, on the one hand, and on the other the responsibilities of managers and commissioners of services to understand and balance the needs of whole populations of users and potential users who might place contrasting demands on services. Finally, as

Holloway points out, those who 'use' the mental health services in the broadest sense are not only those who receive the service but also include their carers and the wider community, whose views might represent quite different interests and concerns, but which also have their legitimate place.

However, in addition to all these legitimate differences of interest and perspective across the spectrum of concerned people, a further theme at this time of great internal change is the existence of less honourable but extremely relevant conflicts of interest. One can hardly fail to notice signs of a battle for control and influence over services between professional groups who feel themselves to be losing power and a newly empowered cadre of service managers. The danger in this is that one or other interest group may seek to represent itself as the users' champion as an astute move in a political struggle. Thus, under the guise of being empowered, the users become the used.

The difficulties attendant on increased user participation in planning groups or the need to take time to obtain users views, can become a convenient scapegoat for failure to make progress. Users can be particularly vulnerable to this sort of scapegoating when they are employed (qua users) as mental health workers. Their roles are often ambiguous, their alliances unclear or fragile and they can easily be held responsible both for not resolving the issue of user empowerment and for being a constant reminder of the difficulty of the task. As the repository of disappointment, guilt and fear users again find themselves disempowered and unable to carry out the functions for which they were employed.

For all that these underlying issues emphasize differences in viewpoint, background and role, it is striking that so many of the contributors to this collection of diverse papers are united in their demonstration of such a substantial degree of personal engagement with the issues and commitment to finding their way through the difficulties. Perhaps the primary value represented in this widespread change in the culture of services is emphasized by Edna Conlan in the first chapter: it is a return to the personal experiences of those suffering mental health problems by all concerned with the issues, not so much to seek directly a solution to the problems of directing and running the services, but as a 'touchstone', a reminder of what lies at their heart. Structures and techniques are means at best: important as they can be these are not what service users are fundamentally looking for. What is sought, perhaps, is an experience of being heard.

Section 1
CONSUMER FEEDBACK AND QUALITY ASSURANCE

1 Consumer feedback: What is useful and acceptable to users

Edna Conlan

This is a personal perspective. I cannot say what is acceptable and useful to all mental health users because, like anyone, we are all different. What I can say something about is what seems to be acceptable and useful for the users that we know and work with in Milton Keynes; I will use that as the context for this paper. One of the problems with that is that Milton Keynes is not typical: it is a new town with new systems in place. We have a district general hospital, an acute unit and a regional secure unit nearby. There is a mental health team in the south of the city and plans for two more; there is a specialist social services mental health team, a team of rehabilitation officers and there are going to be some new creatures called community support officers coming into play. (We were not too enchanted with the advertisement which said they have to be very understanding and able to persuade; we thought: persuade them to do what? Sometimes persuading users to accept what they do not want is at the heart of acceptability).

What kind of service do we really want in Milton Keynes? Has a policy of community care which owes more to the availability of housing in the early years of the new city than to anything else, brought a new world for the user?

We started as an advocacy group in 1987, and I think we were the first advocacy group in the country that looked at both the local hospital and the community. We started a year after the Nottingham Patients' Council Support Group. Two members of the NPCSG came down and we had a wonderful 'empowerment' day which was half users and half professionals. None of us was entirely sure what advocacy meant, and I think we are still unsure because we evolve our own definitions as we go. I think that it is important that what is acceptable and useful to users is the right to define, the right to have people start from where they are.

So where are they in Milton Keynes? There were two large hospitals about 20 miles away in each direction, one is now closed, and although

I am never sure that what we are doing in Milton Keynes is wonderful, I am sure we are doing better than those hospitals. There is more hope, and there is more of a feeling that people are beginning to work together, not just talking about it. Milton Keynes is a new city and wants to be doing the fashionable thing; it wants to be seen to be doing the right thing. (Well, most of it does!)

We have a purpose-built unit which is new (it looks like Lego); we have the single rooms, the four bedded wards, the staff not wearing uniforms – a fairly open place on the whole. But I would not say it is human, and that is what we as users want to find: a place that is human, a place where people are valued. I think that, with all the changes going on at the moment, there is the danger that a whole body of people are being valued because they are a wonderful source of employment over the next few years, a wonderful source of career development. I am not sure that we are any nearer valuing people just because they are people. Sometimes we seem to do it a bit and sometimes we fail; all we know is that it is a long hard struggle.

When the Milton Keynes Advocacy Group started in 1987, we were lucky: we had a Unit General Manager for the mental health services who was quite open minded and let us carry on. The senior nurse manager of the hospital did have worries, but these were focused on what more contact with the mental health services would do to us, not what we might do to them. (I should say that the group is made up of people who are either current users or ex-users of the mental health system. Some are distant users and some of them thought they were distant users, but have not been so in the last year or two – I include myself in that group.)

Doing advocacy work, trying to fight (because it is about fighting in a way, even when it is not adversarial) is not easy. It is stressful, it is tough, you are out on the front line, and sometimes fighting alongside the people you are trying to help. When we first went into our unit, the people we had to convince were the other users: to get them to believe that we were trying to make people understand about quality of life, about improving experience, or about making a service acceptable or useful to them. In our early meetings, what came out most was anger – anger about the things that had happened, about injustice and misunderstandings. That still goes on to some extent, because even when you think you have got a system that is going to work or listen to what people have to say, it is not going to be a perfect system.

I am worried by some other contributions to the discussion of consumer feedback when people talk about the research, talk about satisfaction and so on: there seems to be an assumption that this is a system that works. Four years along the road into advocacy that is still not my understanding. It is my understanding that, like advocacy, sometimes you get it right but more often you get it wrong. Very often the tragedy is that people do not know why they get it wrong. Look at the terminology: 'consumer feedback' is all very well but what about consumer 'satisfaction'? As Ingrid Barker states: 'are we consumers?'. It is like user 'involvement': we have all been involved as users, but how involved can we get the professionals to be? Can we get them involved enough to sit down with us and really listen to what we have to say? The answer to that is sometimes yes and sometimes no. Changes do not come quickly or easily. The awful thing is that sometimes changes you think are going to work (and professionals think are going to work) do not, and you have face the fact that changes do not always work out for the better and that is a hard one to take on board.

Sometimes you have to face the fact that as a user group going in and out and trying to make improvements, you can get it wrong too. You can tread on other people's toes. There has been a question in relation to quality assurance: 'Do people in residential homes want all this intrusion?'. That is a really important question – it is one of the first questions that has to be asked. It is certainly a question that has to be asked if you are an advocate. The first right of a user is the right to tell you that they do not want to know and your job is to respect that: you are not there to push your point of view, or to wave your banner and decide what the orthodox view is.

Over the years user groups have got together and we now have a United Kingdom Advocacy Network. We sometimes think we know what all the issues are and what is important to users, but we do not. One of the things we have learned to do, when we get new members into the group, is to encourage them to speak out when we are asked to train professionals. We can get wheeled on for half an hour to give the user perspective and the professionals are all supposed to be very sympathetic for that time. It can sometimes seem as if we are all going through the motions because including the user perspective is fashionable: it has to be seen to be done. However, you might touch emotion, you might even get people thinking if you involve the new members of the group because of the freshness and directness of each individual's experience. It is not all wasted by any means; some of it is so useful and a real beginning. I have known the ASWs and the CPNs actually to think about what they were doing, to come to terms with or get over their fear of the user movement in those sessions. They are not wasted if they help to change attitudes.

Sometimes when you are trying to consult users, you tend to forget that it is enormously complex. If you are looking at things like consumer satisfaction and so on, you have got to set it in the context of people's lives. You have got to take time to talk to people. You cannot just go into residential homes with a set of questionnaires with your middle class benevolence and kindness and have your half hour interview, even with the best intentions. That is a first step but it is only a beginning. We have got to get to the place where, if you are going to do that, you have got to sit down with some of those users first and get to know them and understand something about their lives. You have to know what they feel like when the benefit book has been taken away, and when they get into hassles with the people who are running the homes because they are at these continual meetings, and their relatives are not allowed to visit because 'we're having a meeting'. You have to understand the flavour of those things. They do not come out in nice little indices: constructs are complicated. Indicators may be helpful. I do not know if we can ever evolve outcome measures. We can evolve something that looks like outcomes and might do for a bit, but that is as much as we can do. We are not going to have perfection; we are not going to have this wonderful world where people are listening and understanding effortlessly. I know that because we have been trying to do it and failing as much as we succeed.

Coming back to Milton Keynes, the Advocacy Group is going in and out of the acute unit, and up to the regional secure unit (one of the few really good ones in the country) regularly. We go to the secure unit on Saturday afternoons. Very often they have birthday parties and dinners and we have a good time there, and we have the people coming to each other's parties from the acute unit and the secure unit. We are changing things – things that might not seem to be to do with consumer feedback or satisfaction and the quality of the service, but have everything to do with people feeling that they might be okay even if they are stuck up there. It is just being able to be together as human beings. It is building a town where the main thing about user involvement is the fact that we begin to care about each other, begin to stand together and be stronger.

In Milton Keynes it is not actually necessary for the advocacy group to go round and tell every user group what to do; they can do that themselves. If they need us, they know where we are and they can come to meetings for a while and get involved, and we are part of the whole structure of users together. It works so much better when you get 2 or 3 people telling you that somebody is in trouble, telling you that they need help and trying to understand how to get it. It is not something you go and tell them, it is something you evolve together; that is what it is about – it is nebulous and it is changing.

This idea of the 'long-term chronically mentally ill': who are these people? These are people away in an institution who have been forced to be long-term mentally ill. They are not the people I know who live in the community who are sometimes ill, sometimes not, sometimes like all of us, make mistakes, stop taking their medication without arranging for supported withdrawal, or take too much. They are people who are genuinely trying to make sense of their lives in their own way. That is something that mental health professionals do not take on board nearly enough, and it is something we have all had to learn about.

There are some interesting papers in this book about the techniques and systems being tried; I do not want to knock them all because I think a lot of those things are really good – Critical Incident Technique, for example. I know that I learned most about Marlborough House when a boy from there jumped off the top of a car park. That for me was a 'critical incident', because the staff, the managers and the users in that secure unit sat there and cried together and wondered how on earth we could have helped. The most poignant thing was that he'd written a poem in the Newsletter just the week before and it was all there. That feeling, that something precious had gone. Maybe we could not have done anything about it but that humanness, feeling, sharing and understanding – that is what consumer satisfaction is really about. It is not about measures, it is not about cleverness, it is about a sense that when you know something is not working for you, you can go and you can talk to somebody and you can get it changed. It may not work but you can try and keep on trying.

The overall impression that often comes across in this area is that users are people who need to be organized; things have to be set up for them. Users are not without resources, and not without ingenuity. Professionals should think on this because they are fairly well paid, and very comfortable. You live for years on benefit and understand what it means to have to buy all your clothes in Oxfam unless a relative gives you something, and how it feels when people up the road treat you as if you are very funny, and you are not sure yourself that you are not very funny. You realize that things are getting on top of you, realize that the world is closing in on you. People with manic depression sometimes say 'My time clock is changing, I know that there's something wrong'. What is important is not taking a doctor's or scientific definition of what mental illness is, but letting people come to an understanding of their own definitions of what it is, and how they can help each other. A group of users like the manic depressive group can sit down and say 'I know I'm going, because of this'. It is these personal resources that users have that need to be understood and respected.

What is useful to us is coming to these understandings about where we are and how we are – not seeing it as a problem that has to be managed, not seeing it as something that has to be made scientific. I know it is about resources, I know it is about costs. I do not think that there is a group of people in the country that know more about resources and costs than mental health patients. We just sit there in some of these waiting rooms and we get treated like shit. We know the costs of being stigmatized as mentally ill. So how do you do anything about that? Something has to be done about those problems. You have to get one

13

world to meet with the other world. I think it is possible, possible to get some complementarity – the inside and outside perspectives giving real depth to understanding the lives of service users.

I do not think that professionals and users have to be shouting at each other. I do not think it is necessary that the outside view and the inside view have to be at war. I think there are possibilities for them to get together but they are enormously complex, and they are going to take sitting down and working out. They are going to be about particular places, particular people – about description as well as explanation. Whether it is about drugs, housing, money or whatever, individual care programmes are first and foremost about individuals. Take that on board, take on that world of difference, take that on when you are designing Case Management schemes and other projects: case management means first of all getting to know people, finding out where they are and engaging with them. It is not going to come out of some preconceived plan – I can't help that, but the act of making real contact can teach an enormous amount about consumer perspectives and about meaningful research which is grounded in social realities.

Users are more likely to respond openly and cooperatively and work with those researchers who focus on the quality of their lives and convey their interest in users as people. Impersonal approaches which have a not too well hidden agenda relating to the efficiency of social control, defending the often indefensible status quo, provide few satisfactions for participating consumers. Kelman (1967) said good research must involve 'the human use of human subjects'. Researchers would do well to remember that objectivity does not mean treating people like objects. That is what is not useful and acceptable to the users I know.

*Reprinted in Bynner & Stribley (eds 1979) Social Research; Principles + Procedures Open UP.

2 Consumer surveys: An overview

Yvonne Webb

Over recent years studies on consumer feedback in mental health services – especially in community mental health centres – have mushroomed, and satisfaction is the most frequently used method of assessment. Despite some tentative 'trends' in findings, for the most part results are often contradictory and confusing. This has not prevented various factions with an interest in mental health issues from using results to support their particular political viewpoint when it suits them. However, it is doubtful whether any firm conclusions can be drawn from present findings, most being 'best described as hypotheses' (Lebow, 1982).

Inconclusive findings are typical of any new area of research, but in this area a lack of commitment in terms of resources and expertise to user research is also to blame. Often mental health professionals are left to find their own means of eliciting user views and in many cases measures are specifically designed for the particular service and setting in which they are administered – there is no generally accepted standard.

Attention to an agreed set of initial problems in consumer research within mental health services would help advance practice and facilitate the development of some general scales. It is also worth identifying those existing instruments which meet some, if not all, of the criteria of acceptable standards of measurement.

This paper will firstly cover some of the apparent trends in published findings; secondly, present the main methodological issues accompanying this type of research; and finally, give some examples of innovatory instruments and approaches to measuring consumer satisfaction within mental health services which can be found in the literature.

An overview of research findings

Emphasis on patient satisfaction with health care services is increasing,

15

particularly in the USA, where community mental health centres are obliged to evaluate their services. However, in many cases, satisfaction measures are designed specifically for the particular service and setting in which they are administered, resulting in a multitude of measures being used, with no generally agreed standard. This has produced limited and frequently conflicting sets of information.

Despite the wide variety of methods used, however, most studies report high levels of satisfaction. These represent impressive although not unanimous levels: Lebow (1982) found that of 63 studies between 54% and 100% of the patients sampled endorsed either in-patient or out-patient settings as generally satisfying.

Critics have consistently used these high levels of satisfaction as evidence that mental health service clients are unable to discriminate between qualitatively different types of service. On the other hand, results have been interpreted to mean that clients are happy with the services that they are receiving, and this has been taken by some to support the view that hospitals, for example, should stay open. Still others contest such findings, arguing that data has been collected without due regard for the complexities of research. Obviously a lot depends on the interpretation of the results of user research, the conclusions drawn, and the implications that these are deemed to have.

Clearly, an important issue is whether satisfaction rates reflect what clients really think of a service. One problem is that, as McIver (1991) argues, clients rarely possess sufficient knowledge of a service to be in a position to compare it with an expected standard; nor is the standard aimed for usually specified to the respondent.

Are existing satisfaction measures sensitive enough to be able to tap into client attitudes? Unfortunately, many early studies have used quite primitive tools, such as single-item measures. As pressure has mounted on services to use satisfaction measures as a method for evaluation, lengthier questionnaires and interviews have been developed which have often been broken down into domains – particularly with the use of factor analysis. Lehman's work (1982) on the measurement of Quality of Life provides one example of this.

Such domains have included satisfaction with staff; recreation; physical surroundings; and specific treatments. Clients have still tended to be satisfied in most areas but with interesting exceptions. They are generally less satisfied with psychiatrists (there tend to be mixed feelings about their usefulness, and psychiatrists are generally less popular than nurses); with medication and the side effects of drugs; with group therapy; and with ward rounds. It is interesting to note that one study found their clients to be more satisfied with doctors than in other studies; the authors suggest this was due to the fact that their clients saw a psychiatrist more, on average, than most clients in mental health services (Piersma, 1987).

What type of questions should be asked? The type of questions included may well have an influence upon levels of satisfaction – particularly if they are relatively superficial questions which have little meaning for clients. Indeed, it has often been found, that providers and users of mental health services do not always agree on the relative importance they assign to various components of satisfaction. (See Elbeck *et al* (1990), for discussion of this issue and a method for eliciting key areas of importance to clients).

It is interesting that more recent studies (perhaps influenced by the user movement and by the human rights movement in general) have begun to include items related to giving information to clients, patient rights and participation in treatment and in management of services with the emerging result that clients are strikingly dissatisfied in these areas (e.g. Macdonald *et al* (1988); GPMH and Camden Consortium (1991); and Hansson (1989)).

One study, for example, found satisfaction to be high with regard to staff – patient relationships, treatment programmes and the physical environment of wards; but low in areas of patient information, influence on management and design of treatment. An overwhelming 82% of clients, for instance, were dissatisfied with existing information about the possibility of reading their case records; over 40% with information about their mental health problems and treatment alternatives; and over half were dissatisfied with the degree of consideration that was given to patients' own views of treatment, and with regard to information about the effects of drugs (Hansson, 1989).

It is also the case that some factors appear to be more important to clients – especially 'human' factors (Raphael, 1972), such as interaction with staff; and particularly the relationship between client and therapist (Hansson (1989); Lee (1979); and Corrigan (1990) who cites a number of studies in this respect). It would be especially useful to discover which satisfaction dimensions are the best predictors; for example, which are the more important dimensions of satisfaction in influencing behaviour? These questions are only now being addressed and remain important issues for future research.

What is the relationship between consumer satisfaction and other outcome measures? Whilst little has been done in this respect, findings indicate that satisfaction is closely related to therapists' assessments of client satisfaction and to clients' global assessments of their success in treatment; but only slightly to therapists' assessment of change. Hansson *et al.* (1989) found that satisfaction was related to clients' self-reported level of global improvement.

To what extent can existing measures predict the behaviour of clients? Most surveys of users of mental health services have used satisfaction as a dependent variable to evaluate provider services and facilities; although of course it can be treated as an independent variable in order to predict consumer behaviour (e.g. use of services). Are satisfied clients, for example, more likely to comply with treatment? In his review, Lebow (1982) failed to find any studies which could report a plausible relationship between reported satisfaction and premature termination. This is an important area, however, as one of the main rationales for consumer research is to make services more acceptable to users, and to encourage better use of services.

Are some clients more likely to be satisfied with services than others? Some studies claim to have found a relationship between one or more demographic factors (e.g. sex, age, race, occupational status, education, etc.) and satisfaction whilst others have found no correlation. There is a similar divergence of opinion in the conclusions of those who have reviewed the literature (e.g. Corrigan (1990) claims to find such a relationship while Weinstein (1981) and Lebow (1982) do not). The widest consensus seems to be, however, that demographic factors are not related to reported satisfaction.

Overall, we have attempted to concentrate here on general agreement between studies. In fact, this might be quite misleading since results from satisfaction studies are more often inconsistent and confusing. The main problem for consumer research in this area is the lack of any standard measures, or even it seems, standards for developing them. With few resources and little in the academic world to draw upon, mental health professionals have been forced to create their own measures of satisfaction. As studies have usually been only concerned with their particular service this has resulted in a multitude of under-developed schedules which have often been put together by a mix and match of previous attempts.

In addition to differences between instruments used to assess satisfaction, there are differences in format (questionnaire or interview); method of contacting respondents; timing of the assessment; the extent to which non-respondents are followed up and so on. It is useful, therefore, to identify the methodological issues that should be addressed by those who are attempting to elicit user views.

Methodological issues

It might be worth pointing out first that **any** research is subject to problems and that the subject matter of this particular research should not be seen as the overriding obstacle to success. The fact that such research has often not been pursued with as much rigour as other types is, in part, a reflection of the status that has been attached to its importance in the evaluation of mental health services. It must be remembered that a greater financial commitment buys more experienced research staff and the time and expertise, therefore, for a more sophisticated study. Meanwhile, consumer research in this field is in the very early stages of development and we should aim to encourage this development rather than be put off by what amounts to merely the normal process of scientific investigation.

Nonetheless, underlying any use of satisfaction data is the assumption that satisfaction questionnaires reliably and accurately measure client satisfaction. Unfortunately, many studies have been undertaken without proper regard for good measurement practices. It is therefore worth going over some of the methodological problems which, if not taken into account, are likely to cast doubt on findings.

Appropriate **sampling** of respondents is necessary. For the purpose of accurate measurement it is unfortunate that unsatisfied customers will be most likely to drop out of the service and so be less accessible for inclusion in a survey. To deal with this problem some surveys have concentrated on the opinions of new contacts or first admissions. Practical sampling concerns have also involved the exclusion of those who refuse or do not respond; those for whom the involvement would be an undue source of stress; and clients who are considered to be too disabled to be able to give meaningful responses (although some have tackled this problem by using relatives or guardians).

Lebow (1982) reports, for example, studies which suggest that non-respondents differ from respondents in ways that are likely to affect reports of satisfaction, and that these differences are not demographic ones but treatment characteristics. This is worth bearing in mind when studies present data on non-respondents.

What **method** should be used? Weinstein (1981) argues in a rather polemical paper that, as far as in-patient studies are concerned, quantitative studies have revealed higher levels of satisfaction than qualitative studies carried out in the 60s and 70s which relied on interviews with selected individuals or upon the investigators masquerading as patients.

Weinstein concludes that 'the defenders of mental hospitals have more accurately portrayed the patients' view'. However, it cannot be assumed that high levels of satisfaction reflect the feelings of patients more accurately; indeed given their generally poor surroundings it seems rather strange that patients should be so happy with their lot – prompting many to doubt the sensitivity of the research schedules being used. It is probably the case moreover, that a questionnaire format has been selected as an approved method for enquiries about fairly cosmetic aspects of the patient's care such as the quality of food, cleanliness of wards, and so on, which, whilst clearly important, probably stir feelings less deeply than say, the way the patient is treated as a person during his or her stay. Interviews are more likely to rouse strong feelings and possibly less positive ones; and are also often selected for this very reason. It must be accepted therefore that the selection and composition of a certain method will almost certainly reflect the researcher's bias towards a particular kind of result. It is perhaps telling that the studies were unable to differentiate between hospitals; nor did levels of satisfaction alter much over long periods of time when they would have been expected to improve with more progressive policies over the years.

Thus it is likely that both qualitative and quantitative methods used side by side will generate the most interesting and valid results. Efforts can also be made to increase the objectivity of qualitative methods, for example by getting verbatim comments from a representative sample of respondents and not just those who volunteer them, or those who are the most articulate. Additionally, as McIver (1991) points out, there may be a need to use different methods for different types of client. For example, it is only appropriate to use the self-completion questionnaire if all of the potential respondents can see, read English, use their hands, and can understand and feel comfortable with this particular method.

Either way, consideration must also be given to the **problems of each method:** reactivity threatens validity where the respondent answers in a way that s/he thinks the interviewer or researcher would like; or when influenced by the interviewer's characteristics in some way. This is particularly a problem for people with mental health problems who often suffer low self-esteem as a result of the adverse effects that mental illness has had on their lives including stigma, unemployment, poverty, and loss of valued roles.

It is far preferable that an independent researcher or professional administer questionnaires or interviews and not a person who is directly involved in the client's care. Most importantly the respondent must be ensured confidentiality – fear of reprisal will seriously inflate satisfaction scores, for no matter how dissatisfied a client may be, in the context of few alternatives to conventional patterns of care, they are not likely to risk losing the only service available to them if there is a perceived risk of personal identification.

Some researchers now ask users first what they expect from mental health services or whether any particular elements of the service have been particularly important in their care. It is worth aiming for only the important domains and therefore keeping the measure fairly short and 'user friendly' (i.e. easy to respond to, problems of acquiescence and reactivity withstanding).

A further issue concerns the meaning of the terms used. Such terms as satisfied, very satisfied and helped mean different things to different individuals (Lebow, 1982). For example, to some, satisfaction means a minimum state of acceptability of services, whereas for others it means near perfection. The inclusion of more questions or definitions can help this problem. Furthermore, as McIver (1991) argues, if the concept of satisfaction is used this too often assumes that patients possess a sufficient knowledge of services to compare them with adequate alternatives. It should be made clear to respondents the standards which are aimed for and quite specific questions aimed at monitoring these standards should be asked. Another difficulty lies in the inclusion of items concerned with non-satisfaction. There is nothing wrong with instruments with mixed items so long as they are kept conceptually separate. A number of studies, however, assume inaccurately that positive responses to non-satisfaction items indicate satisfaction.

Another major concern is that of the **reliability** of scales which has often not been reported. Although reliability issues have been addressed by more recent studies, as Lebow (1982) points out it is precisely those studies that are methodologically suspect for which reliability is unknown. Single item measures are less reliable than scales, whilst lengthy, homogeneous scales are likely to be the most reliable (Ware *et al*, 1978).

Designs and analyses have tended to be fairly simplistic in many studies, and the presentation of method and results has also been poor. At a minimum, a report should be absolutely clear about the precise purpose and aims of the study, including specific details about the method used – items omitted are often the most important, eg response rate, criteria for assessment and ethical procedures. Further, each report should at least indicate the degree of satisfaction in terms of both means and standard deviation and the frequencies of consumers responding at various levels of satisfaction (Lebow, 1982). Only with such information is the reader in an adequate position to begin to make sense of the results reported.

In summary, questionnaires and interviews often look deceptively simple. It may only be when embroiled in the design of a study that the real difficulties become clear. Oppenheim's (1966) book remains one of the best guides to questionnaire design. Furthermore, issues about the organization and implementation of a survey need to be addressed at the very beginning: objectives, resources, implementation (including pilot studies and reliability and validity tests), coding, using statistics and report-writing. The International Hospital Federation management handbook, *And What Would They Know About It?* (1988) is of considerable use for preparatory work. Above all, user research deserves the same respect as any other type of scientific research. This means not just in terms of attention to the findings, but in careful attention by the investigators to methodological issues from the start.

Satisfaction measures – what is available?

There are numerous satisfaction schedules available which have been developed in response to practical evaluation programmes for specific settings. It is therefore difficult to use any of these without some modification, and of course this is what usually happens; people use various bits of other questionnaires for their own purposes with a multitude of hybrids as a result, very few of which have been adequately tested.

It is very difficult to find any widely used questionnaires or interviews which can act as a standard and which meet the criteria for scientifically acceptable measures. It would be a worthwhile future task to produce a guide to what is available and to document the relative attributes each measure has to offer. Meanwhile there are one or two schedules of interest from the literature which are worth describing briefly here, although not an exhaustive list nor even a representative sample of the available instruments.

In terms of **identifying components** for satisfaction there are two recent studies which address this issue. The first, by Elbeck *et al* (1990) used a focus-group method to generate attributes of ideal care from the patient's viewpoint. The authors found that, from a number of items, two factors emerged; these were associated with behavioural autonomy and supportive care. It was found, in fact, that supportive care was by far of most concern to patients. This area included items such as positive interpersonal support from staff and particularly from the client's psychiatrist. These findings support those from other authors such as Raphael (1972), Gordon (1979) and Weinstein (1981) who have also found interpersonal relationships with staff to be important to clients.

The second study is by Waismann and Rowland (1989) who designed an instrument for use with people with a chronic, potentially long-term mental illness. In fact, the instrument can be used with anyone (including people who do not suffer from mental health problems). This involved a fixed choice card-sorting format which enables clients to rate the importance of 10 areas of need associated with stress and distress. Six factors were shown to be of particular importance: recreation, finance, household, occupational role, safety and accommodation. It has also been used to rate satisfaction with aspects of the service although the results of this have yet to be reported.

Probably the most well-known measure for **in-patients** is Raphael's (1972) questionnaire which was administered to 2,148 in-patients resident in nine hospitals between 1970 and 1971. This study can be seen as an important landmark along the road of user research, not least because of the relatively huge sample size. The questionnaire itself has since been widely used. It should be borne in mind, however, that this questionnaire does not rate satisfaction as such on all items but rather asks patients to choose from a series of Yes/No responses concerning the favourableness of certain aspects of the hospital. There are also some weaknesses in its design – mainly to do with its simplicity. McIver (1991) usefully suggests ways to overcome these weaknesses in her practical guide to user research in mental health services. For example, she points out that Raphael's questions appear to have been set by service providers and points to previous research which has explored the aspects of service provision which users consider to be important. McIver also notes that the Raphael questionnaire covers a wide range of topics with very few questions, and suggests ways to gather more in-depth information around each topic. An alternative in-patient questionnaire is PATSAT developed by CASPE **in West London** on general medical care, but which is now being adapted for use in mental health services. (See Heckels, Chapter 3).

A measure from America called the Satisfaction With Mental Health Care Scale (SMHCS) (Slater *et al*, 1982) fills the gap in relation to **outpatient services** and constitutes one of the few satisfaction tools to fulfil psychometric requirements including reliability, validity and factor analysis. The questionnaire consists of 32 items based on a Likert scale of 'strongly agree – strongly disagree', and is completed by clients. It has not yet been tested on in-patients although there were plans to do so at the time of publication.

Again, there are a number of measures available which have been used for very specific purposes. As its name suggests, however, the General Satisfaction Questionnaire has been marketed for use in a variety of settings and with different client populations. The GSQ, designed by Huxley *et al* (1980) at Manchester University, has recently been tested both here and in the USA within CMHCs, day centres, sheltered work settings, and in hospitals. From the results it appears to have some face validity, and in responding to it clients have discriminated between items. It was also interesting to observe in the results a major difference between UK clients' reported satisfaction and that of clients in the USA, the latter being much more dissatisfied with services. The uncertainty about how to interpret this result – is it differences in services or in cultural norms? – is typical of the field. Unfortunately, results have not yet been published on reliability and validity, although there are plans to do so.

Conclusions

There are many conflicting – not to mention dubious – findings within the literature, although some tentative 'trends' might be elicited. Many problems, however, could be overcome by more sophisticated research methods, but this demands that more commitment in terms of time, resources, and expertise be given to user research. It is essential that we gain the consumer's view of mental health services. As Lebow (1982) points out: 'In so far as treatment cannot occur without the willingness of the client to participate in sessions, minimal satisfaction is a necessary condition for treatment success'.

Illustrating the significance of this issue, in a recent service activity project (Clifford and Webb, 1991) which involved a survey of the characteristics and patterns of service use of 2,149 clients in acute psychiatric care, professionals reported that: of 1,699 clients, 533 did not always take the medication prescribed to them; 848 out of 2,070 did not always meet appointments with their therapist; and 229 out of 1,005 were prone to abruptly ceasing contact with the service. 742 clients out of 2,136 displayed either a mixed or definitely negative attitude towards the service that they were receiving. It is important to bear in mind that this was only the professionals' point of view and could be a significant underestimate, as professionals may be reluctant to report that clients are not happy with their service.

Finally, the manner in which 'satisfaction' research is undertaken must constantly be borne in mind. It is easy to charge in on clients with a questionnaire or interview and charge out again. Care must be taken that the research is not invasive; and to ensure that the clients are thoroughly informed from the start and that they receive feedback on the results. Indeed, perhaps we should get to know better the clients we are asking to help us, and the types of lives they lead, as well as pursuing fairly limited information through the means of structured questionnaires or interviews.

This raises the question of what measuring satisfaction actually means both to clients and researchers, as well as to clinicians and managers of services. Is it enough to ask about satisfaction – or should we also be employing methods of obtaining the users' views which are more inclusive and meaningful for the respondent?

3 Obtaining the customer's view using the CASPE patient satisfaction system

Victoria Heckels

Interest in measuring patient satisfaction in the Health Service has greatly increased in recent years. 'Working for Patients' (HMSO, 1989), emphasized the need to monitor that services meet patients' requirements and to ensure that patients' views of the quality of services are considered by those providing their care. The feedback from patients of their perception of the quality of services received should affect the activities of both purchasers and providers, and the quality factor could become an important factor affecting the demand for services. There is no reason why mental health services should be excluded from these new expectations.

As a result of these changes, managers now require information on patient satisfaction of a kind which can help them make informed decisions on the consumers' behalf. This creates a need to develop a method of obtaining and monitoring patients' views which would cover all aspects of patients care. Managers need a tool which is sensitive enough not only to measure patient satisfaction but also to monitor the subsequent success of any changes made.

This paper describes how the CASPE system has been used to measure patient satisfaction in psychiatric hospitals, why such research is required, and potential problems of working in this area. The research reported has been mainly funded by the Department of Health.

The CASPE system in general hospital care

The CASPE patient satisfaction system was originally designed to measure and monitor continuously the levels of satisfaction of acute hospital medical and surgical patients with all aspects of their care and also to facilitate the use of information to improve services so as to ensure patients' satisfaction. Particular emphasis is placed by CASPE on continuous monitoring since previous studies (e.g. Hyde-Price, 1986) have shown that one-off surveys tend to be ignored by managers. In contrast, research on the CASPE in-patients questionnaire has shown that executive action is more likely to be taken if managers receive patients' views on a regular basis (Wickings *et al*, 1989). The continuous monitoring provided by the CASPE system is intended to promote a consumer orientation among professional and other staff, unit managers and purchasers.

Initial development of the CASPE system took place in Bloomsbury Health Authority and the DoH subsequently considered it important to validate the system in other health districts. Six were selected to give a reasonable cross-section of sizes and types of District Health Authorities in the NHS and subsequently many more hospitals have started to use the system. During the evaluation research, patient satisfaction questionnaires were distributed routinely to acute in-patients; acute out-patients; ante-natal and post-natal, obstetrics in- and out-patients.

The emphasis was on the construction of self-completion questionnaires constructed in as simple and clear a format as possible. A four-point Likert 'smiley faces' scale (very dissatisfied, somewhat dissatisfied, satisfied, very satisfied) has proved to be readily understandable and to give results that are sensitive to change. This satisfaction scale is rated in relation to sixteen broad topics developed from structured interviews with patients. The process of deriving and revising these topics can be undertaken anew for other specialties. The approach is therefore a very flexible one. Subsequent work has expanded the application of the patient satisfaction systems into many other areas of hospital care. These include acute psychiatry, paediatrics, accident and emergency, genitourinary medicine services and intensive care patients.

It is crucial to the thinking behind the CASPE approach that it can be simply integrated with the routine management information systems already in place. This results in a cost-effective approach to regular monitoring. There are three CASPE systems that can be used: a computerized version, a manual version and a stand-alone software model. The first and most versatile is the computerized version. The way the system works in practice for General Hospitals is best illustrated by a flow diagram (see Figure 1).

Patient details such as name, sex and ward are entered on the hospital's computerized patients administration system. The patient satisfaction system (PATSAT) takes these details and 'downloads' them to a PC. The software can then generate a questionnaire identified only by code which is in turn sent to the ward or clinic, with a personalized letter asking each patient to complete the questionnaire. These are returned anonymously in sealed envelopes (preserving confidentiality of opinions from clinical staff).

Questionnaires are designed to make scoring of large numbers a simple, mechanical task. The patients' responses are read by an Optical Mark Reader at CASPE, and the collated response data is used to produce

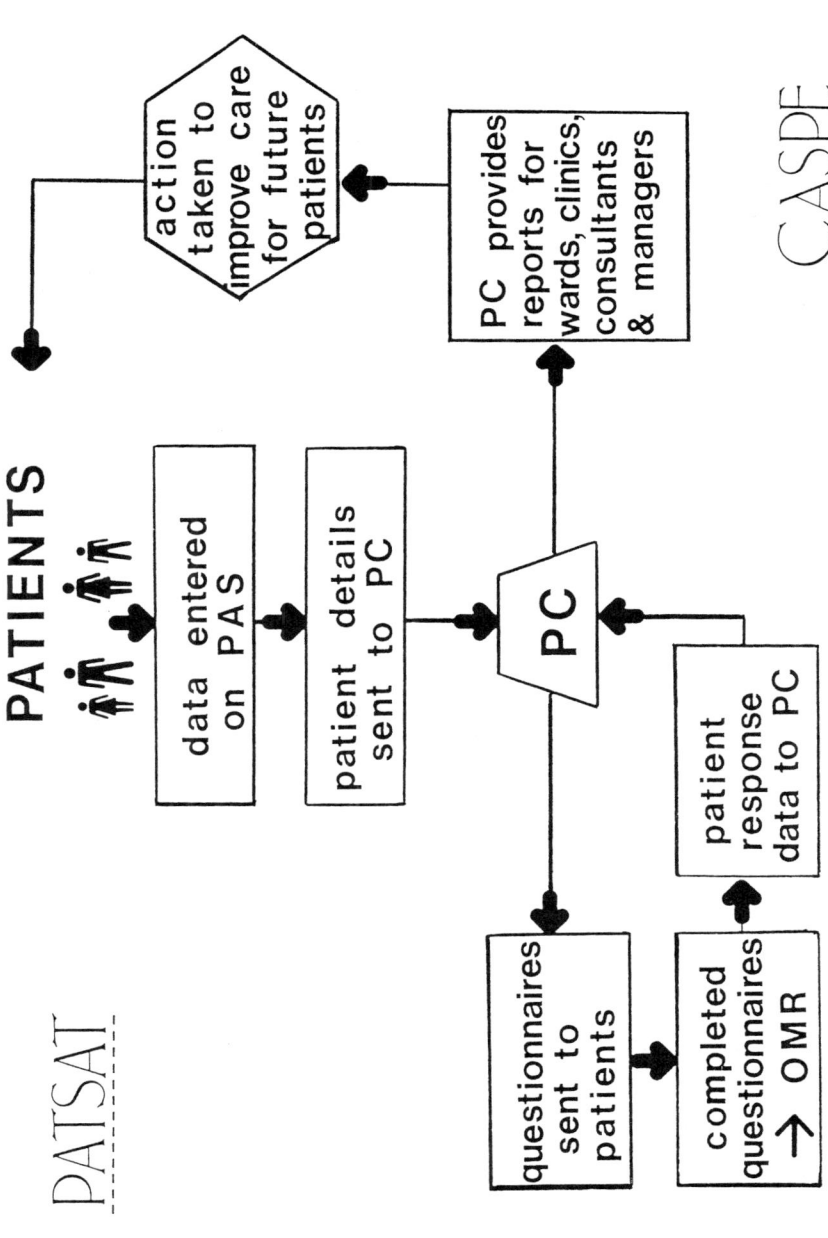

Figure 1 Computerized CASPE System

27

reports providing indices of patient satisfaction overall and with each of the selected topics at ward and clinic level, and for consultants and managers. This information should enable action to be taken to improve the care of future patients.

The second system is known as the non-PAS or manual system. This was developed to take account of those health authorities that do not have certain specialties or out-patients' data on their PAS. This means that the completed questionnaires cannot be linked to patients. Consequently this limits the reporting facility and reports can only be aggregated to a distribution point, such as a ward, clinic consultant or specialty. The third system is known as the Survey model. This is a stand-alone software model which was developed so that questionnaires can be used in areas where it is not possible or practical to download data or pre-code questionnaires.

Other features of the questionnaire

As well as including standard core questions in all sites, the questionnaires have the facility to include up to eleven additional topics which are selected by local managers. As examples, the local 'management-driven' topics appearing on the pilot psychiatric questionnaire have included 'the information given about your condition', 'the amount of time spent with your doctor' and 'the access you have to telephones'.

The core topics are very general and are intended to highlight broad areas of concern and monitor them over time. However, when dissatisfaction occurs, it is important for managers to know the precise reason for it. If this is not immediately obvious, **subsidiary questionnaires** are available, which provide a more in-depth analysis. These second-level questionnaires are intended to be a 'snapshot' focusing on a particular area of service. This type of questionnaire uses an attitude scale that ranges from 'I strongly agree' to 'I strongly disagree'. The questions are phrased either positively or negatively in order to assess the strength of patients' opinions and to help control for response bias.

The main top-level in-patient, post-natal and ante-natal questionnaires have been **translated** into six different languages: Bengali, Chinese, Greek, Gujarati, Turkish, and Yiddish. These questionnaires can be held on the wards for staff to hand out when necessary. Patients are informed that they are available via a translated message printed on the reverse of the English questionnaire.

The **reporting formats** should be flexible enough to meet the needs of all levels in the organization, from ward level to General Manager. The information is available as graphical reports and information can be aggregated by ward, clinic, specialty, consultant and hospital, or by Health Authority purchaser, contract or GP Fund Holder. Managers can either look at all the topics on the questionnaire, a selection of them, or just one. At present the routine reports of the patients' satisfaction are produced for managers. These reports either use index figures or percentages to calculate the satisfaction levels. Because the PATSAT system is linked to the hospital PAS, the satisfaction scores can be further analysed by any information held on the PAS. This means that information can also be reported by ward and consultant, as well as by age, sex and postcode.

In addition to the questionnaires patients are asked whether they would like to make **additional comments**. They often accept this opportunity, especially as their anonymity is guaranteed. The comments are typed by topic into a software package called Asksam which is a text storage and retrieval system. This means that additional reports can be produced from verbatim comments made by patients. Information can be stored and reproduced at any time and in any format that managers feel appropriate for their needs.

Areas of patients' dissatisfaction should stimulate **management action**. Sometimes these actions may only be minimal changes which are, nonetheless, important to patients. More significant changes may take longer to achieve. In order to improve the quality of care, standards can be set (in terms of satisfaction indices and proportion of dissatisfied respondents) which illustrate to managers and other staff whether the levels of patient satisfaction they achieve are adequate. When standards are not met by current data returns corrective management action should be automatically triggered. Thus, the **continuous monitoring** of satisfaction on a regular, routine basis rather than occasional, one-off exercises is central to the CASPE system. Standards can be changed over time to seek an improved quality of care.

Previous research into psychiatric patients' attitudes

After the hospitals' system had been developed for most acute services, research was undertaken in psychiatry. The published literature appears to show that, although the need to sample user opinion on most psychiatric wards on a regular basis had been recognized (Shields, Morrison and Hart, 1988), work seeking psychiatric patients' views about their treatment and care was limited.

The lack of interest may be due to a number of reasons:

- There is a false perception that psychiatric illness renders patients unable to make valid comments about what happens to them (Shields, 1985);

- NHS psychiatric facilities serve a high proportion of financially disadvantaged and socially rejected individuals who may not have the resources to seek alternative care. These patients are powerless if they are dissatisfied with the services they receive (Holcomb *et al*, 1989);

- Some observers claim that institutional care can result in a lower concern for the patient's welfare than staff's 'prerogatives and role status' (Shields, 1985).

However there are a number of reasons why psychiatric patients' views on their care and treatment should be sought. First, for people in long-stay care, the quality of care may be synonymous with the quality of life. Second, patients' views may help to provide the most effective care possible. Third, ordinary citizens should be empowered as far as possible (Pugh, 1990).

Previous studies have reported that there are many areas of patients' dissatisfaction with mental health care. The Camden Consortium (1989) found that psychiatric patients complained that, around the time of admission, the staff were so concerned with administrative requirements that they were unable to discuss patients' illness. Patients felt that the waiting time for admission was too long and that too little information was given to them about the structure of the hospital. While in hospital they were sometimes frightened by other patients, while staff ignored any conflicts between patients. Physical surroundings were another source of complaint. Levels of noise were heavily criticized – including that from other patients and that from the TV and radio. Patients said they could not sleep at night because of the noise.

In an earlier study, Raphael *et al* (1977) found areas of patient dissatisfaction with the lack of privacy, too few chairs in the dayroom and overcrowding in the dormitories. Patients suggested that they should have the choice of single rooms or shared dormitories. Patients also complained about the lack of privacy in the washrooms, bathrooms and toilets, insufficient storage for personal belongings, no keys for their lockers and that telephone calls could not be confidential.

Shields *et al* (1988) found there was dissatisfaction with food quality, variety and temperature, and inappropriate special diets. The Camden Consortium (1989) heard other complaints about food including stodginess, lack of choice, shortage of fresh fruit, salads and vegetables, insufficient time to eat, and the fact that staff ate separately.

In Shields *et al*'s study (1989), patients wanted more information about how the ward was organized, for instance, covering meal times and shop hours. Patients also felt insufficiently informed about their own treatment and wanted more information about their drugs. They said that usually no alternative treatments were offered and no explanation of the drugs' benefits or side effects was given to them. Complaints were made about the lack of contact with doctors, with a desire to see consultants more often.

Pilgrim and Rogers (1990) found that patients said they were not offered alternatives to hospital admission. Some were not informed of their diagnosis or given reasons for their detainment. Patients claimed that no alternatives to drug treatment were given, and that they were given major tranquillizers without consent. Boredom was another major complaint, especially at weekends.

Shields *et al* conclude that it is necessary to involve psychiatric patients in studies concerning their care. This is especially true in the light of Mayer and Rosenblatt's (1974) finding that staff and patients have different views on what are the most important aspects of care. The CASPE project set out to design a questionnaire which would routinely provide the patients' views.

The CASPE system in acute psychiatric in-patient services

In adapting the CASPE approach to make it applicable to patients in acute psychiatric services we have drawn on these substantive findings from previous research but more heavily upon an empirical process of development in this area. The questionnaire has been designed to include only those topics identified by patients as being most important to them. This approach to questionnaire development can be divided into three phases.

Initially an open-ended structure is used in face-to-face interviews with acute psychiatric in-patients. These interviews are used to identify those aspects of care which patients judge to be most important. Patients are also asked more specific questions relating to topics which had been identified in previous studies. These questions are included so that if a particular topic arose from the open-ended questions, the patient would be prompted to provide additional explanations which will help in the wording of questions. However, answers to these prompted questions are not included in the assessment of what has priority for patients. (A representative sample of patients is obtained to ensure that results are not biased).

A pilot questionnaire is then developed on the basis of the topics raised during interviewing in the first phase. Topics are ranked according to the number of patients who refer to them. This analysis of the issues raised by patients determines the questions appearing on a pilot questionnaire. The questionnaire was then piloted on the acute wards of two psychiatric hospitals, using volunteer patients only. An in-depth interview with the patients was conducted after they had completed the pilot questionnaire to test its validity, i.e. to ensure that there was a correspondence between the researchers' and the patients' interpretation of each question. The precise wording of the questions was also validated, and amended if necessary.

In phase three the questionnaire was piloted for three months and was designed to test the logistics of using a questionnaire to measure and monitor the patients' opinions of psychiatric services. The pilot was also used to determine the best method of delivering the questionnaires to patients.

The results of the pilot suggest that the non-PAS (manual) version was a more appropriate method of questionnaire distribution for this group and that questionnaire distribution should be incorporated into the discharge procedure.

Conclusion

The research project aimed to discover whether the CASPE system is appropriate for this patient group and if it is, to determine the best method of using the questionnaires. The response rate during the piloting of the questionnaire was low. A number of difficulties were identified including the timing of handing the questionnaire out; the duration of the patient's illness; the patient throughput.

Some discussion took place as to whether it is useful to have a questionnaire approach with these difficulties. On balance it was felt the system should continue. With such a disadvantaged group, any means that can be used for them to express their views should be harnessed and the procedural problems need to be ironed out by the management.

4 User input into Total Quality Management: The Critical Incident Technique

Lyn Jones

Introduction

This is a straightforward account of a particular way of getting and making use of service users' views. When I first used this approach it was at someone else's instigation and I was not entirely convinced that it was valid, or would have any impact. Neither, on the other hand, did I believe it would be fruitless – I was reasonably open-minded and happy to give it a try. Since then I have carried out four such exercises, two of them in Mental Health Units, and I feel much more positive about the method. I am not yet an evangelist for the approach, but I do see many merits in it, and it definitely deserves to be presented to and debated by all those concerned with improving health services.

What will be described in this chapter is a means of getting users' views about services as part of a Total Quality Programme. A Total Quality Programme is a management initiated drive to reorient the attention and motivation of staff: to get them to lever themselves out of the ruts of methods, routines, attitudes in which they may have been stuck and take a fresh look at what they are doing. The focus of this fresh look is Quality: the quality of service each member of staff gives to the ultimate service users. In the current language of management, its objective is a culture change.

A crucial early stage in most such programmes is getting a broad cross-section of views about how good the current quality of service is. These views come from users and staff (mainly grassroots staff), with users in a majority. This is done – in this case – using a particular semi-structured interview technique called the Critical Incident Technique, which will be described below.

This chapter therefore addresses, though it does not pretend to answer, two questions:

- Can users' views be put across effectively in the context of a management-initiated, management-controlled programme like a Total Quality Programme?

- Is the Critical Incident Technique an effective and valid method of gathering users' views?

Total Quality Programmes: the current management thinking

The general aim of Total Quality Programmes is as outlined briefly above. The general assumptions behind them are of a kind that have gained widespread currency in management circles over the last few years. These can be summarized very broadly as follows:

- successful organizations place quality at the forefront of their consciousness;

- good quality can only be achieved if all members of the organization are motivated to work for it;

- the key judge of quality is the 'customer' – the person who receives the goods or services provided.

It is not necessary to elaborate further for the present purpose, except to point out that the term 'customer' is used in a very general sense. There are all those outside the organization for whom it supplies goods or services – the 'customers', in the usual sense – plus perhaps others who might be affected by the organization's activities. In the context of mental health services, these external customers might include not only 'patients' but those in a caring relationship to them. Then there are all those inside the organization who consume each others' services. For example, in a hospital the works department rarely has a direct service relationship with the ultimate 'external' customer; it supplies services to 'internal customers', such as ward sisters or catering staff, to enable them in turn to serve the end user. Practically all staff, in this sense, are 'internal customers' of each other's services. However, among different varieties of 'customer', the one which has primacy is the end user.

Total Quality Programmes based on this approach were first instituted in the Scottish Health Service two or three years ago. A couple of programmes were contracted out to management consultants; later the Management Development Group developed its own version, which it has now applied to several Health Board Units in Scotland.

The Management Development Group (MDG) is part of the Common Services Agency of the Scottish Health Service. It provides management education, training and development in various forms to Health Boards and Units in Scotland, sometimes directly, sometimes by bringing in outside resources. Its staff act as internal 'management consultants'; their clients are usually the management of a Health Service Unit, or equivalent. The MDG consultants suggest a programme of action which they discuss with the management of the Unit and adapt as necessary. Their suggested programme is quite complex in detail but has three key elements:

- gaining commitment to the idea of quality as a guiding principle, by involving a broad management team;

- getting data on current quality from 'the customers';

- formulating and implementing a programme of action based on this data.

These three elements are applied first of all with a management team at the most senior level, usually an expanded Unit Management Team, which the MDG calls the 'Top Team'. Then they are replicated one level down, within Departments, and possibly further, with the intention that the ideas and momentum will 'cascade' down the organization. This might well entail further programmes of consumer feedback of a more specific and detailed kind. This chapter, however, concerns only the gathering of data for the Top Team phase.

Scottish Health Feedback has evolved from some years of exploration into how the views of health service users might best be gathered and deployed. This took place at first within a University context – the Department of Community Medicine at Edinburgh University – but since December 1990 Scottish Health Feedback has become an independent organization, charging for its services. It undertakes survey work of various kinds, as well as consultancy in the field of consumer feedback. Scottish Health Feedback was approached by the Management Development Group to organize the interviewing for its Total Quality programmes, for its main 'data collection' phase – the second of the three key elements described above. This partnership has now been working in four units, including two Mental Health Units, with others in the pipeline.

Data collection in the Total Quality process

The main data collection phase – that is, the gathering of views of users and staff about current service quality – comes very early on in the process, just after the Top Team has been formed, but before it has defined which areas of activity will claim its attention. This, in fact, is the principal function of the data collection – to provide a solid basis for the

Top Team to draw up its agenda. This means that the way opinions are gathered must fulfil certain criteria:

- it must allow respondents themselves to define what are the areas of concern;

- it must cover as much of the unit's activities as possible, which means a broad scatter of respondents;

- the views should be collected in a form that can be processed by the management team, not by an outside agency, so that the agenda is defined by those who will have to pursue it.

The views gathered, then, are the start of a process, not the end of it. They do not of themselves define where action is needed; they provide evidence, not judgements. In particular, statistical processing and reasoning would be quite out of place. It is quite inappropriate to form quasi-scientific conclusions. This an awareness-raising activity – broad and systematic, but not quantitative. Finally, one more requirement needs to be observed. It is as important that the process should identify areas of good practice as areas of poor practice. Good practice needs to be reinforced and extended, not forgotten or undervalued.

In each of the projects undertaken so far we have arranged 500 interviews, typically consisting of 250 patients, 50 visitors/relatives and 200 staff. We employ a team of 4 or 5 trained interviewers, working over 4 to 6 weeks. Interviewees are selected, as far as possible, at random; one major but unavoidable restriction on this is that we have to take clinical advice, usually from a charge nurse or equivalent, about who is well enough to be approached.

The interviews follow a semi-structured format. The aim is to identify incidents of behaviour which the respondent has experienced personally, and which he or she thinks are examples of good quality or poor quality service. After a brief introduction, the interviewer asks a suitable general question, leaving quite open what area of service the response might concern. If the respondent gives an example, the interviewer elicits sufficient concrete information to describe the essentials of the 'incident', then asks for more examples. If examples are slow in coming, the interviewer uses a second general question, then moves on to a series of prompts which direct attention to the major areas of experience with the service that the respondent might have.

The interviewer takes brief notes as the interview proceeds. As soon as possible thereafter she transcribes the notes on to separate sheets. Each sheet contains one example of an incident or behaviour, described briefly in the respondent's own words (as closely as the interviewer can recall). Most descriptions are between two and six lines long. Out of the 500 interviews, between 1,800 and 2,600 such 'incident sheets' are produced. These must then be 'processed'.

They are presented, as they stand, to the Top Team formed by the Unit Management. As mentioned above this team is typically the Unit Management Team augmented by further key senior personnel to include 16 to 20 people in total. Doctors, nurses and paramedical staff are prominent in the membership. The processing of the data takes 2 – 3 days of this team's time – a major commitment in itself. The first day is taken up mainly with reading the sheets (in groups of three or four), and sorting and re-sorting them into categories that make sense to the team members. The remainder of the time is taken up identifying programmes of action for each of the areas of concern emerging from this categorization. A set of objectives is drawn up, a deadline agreed and a member of the team nominated to be responsible for taking action.

The day during which the incidents are read and categorized is an interesting one to observe. Relatively little goes on overtly; there is a lot to be read, and groups are silent much of the time as they read each sheet and put it on to a pile. The silence is broken by queries to colleagues about how to categorize an incident, by laughter and the reading out of some description which has amused the reader; by occasional discussion about the definition of categories. Sometimes someone reads out a particularly telling observation or critical response; or a heartfelt compliment. What is notable by its absence is any open attempt to devalue or discredit the responses. The verbatim descriptions carry a great weight of down-to-earth validity which is difficult to gainsay – at least in the context of the team meeting.

The conversation in breaks tends to confirm this impression. Members are, in my opinion, usually pleased and surprised by the volume of compliments: the appreciative comments are usually in the majority. As far as negative comments go, people rarely confess to surprise: the Unit's deficiencies, they say, are well known to them. I think – but have no way to confirm – that there is more to it than that. It is one thing to be aware at some level, of deficiencies, and another to have them documented in concrete detail; I suspect that a good deal of private mental adjustment goes on, and that these vignettes also start off a social process of absorption and interpretation, too subtle to observe from outside.

It is possible to build up a rich and complex picture of what goes on from the thousands of comments collected. Some examples will help to illustrate this. Here, then, are some positive comments:

One of the nurses introduced me to the other patients on my first day here.

There's nothing bad about here. It has helped me a lot. The nursing staff and doctors know when I need to come in and they bring me in. This is my 14th time. It's tremendous. They are always there when I need them and it's the security of knowing that, that keeps me calm.

I was allowed to go to the [General] Hospital to see my mother. This was very imporant to me and I was very pleased about going. I think they'd let me go again if I need to.

I've been here a week and have asked to go on different medication when I saw the doctor. I then saw the charge nurse and was told that my request is being looked into. So, I was taken seriously.

These are typical of the level of comment, mostly straightforward and practical, each not particularly striking but significant as part of an overall picture.

As mentioned earlier, there is a well-documented reluctance among health service users of all sorts to express criticisms. The negative comments, therefore, are of particular interest. When a respondent makes a negative comment, the interviewer follows up with a question about whether the respondent has done anything about the problem, and if not, why not; and then asks, further, whether the respondent has any suggestions for improvement. Here are some examples of negative comments and responses to these supplementary questions:

It's very boring here. There's nothing to do, not a thing.

[Suggestions for improvement?] Why not open up the leisure room at night? This would take some of the tension off.

Nurses should be taking patients on outings into town if they suffer from panic attacks. They won't get better sitting on the ward. They need to build up their confidence outside.

The TV is never off. It's on first thing in the morning. Some people are deaf so it's up loud. I hate it. It's so noisy here – no quietness.

I don't like the atmosphere here. I can't explain it very well but the nurses and patients don't always get on. There's always some person getting on to you to do this or that.

[Did the respondent do anything?] I just keep my mouth shut. It's best to.

The unit sitting room is for patients. I like to go there for peace. The back shift, however, come in there to eat before they come on at 2pm and so they can watch 'Neighbours' and they throw me out. They also smoke in what is supposed to be a non-smoking room.

[Did the respondent do anything?]D'you want me transferred out? If I say any more, I'll be out.

I've been here six weeks. Both times I have seen the consultant, he has had five or six other people in the room, students, social worker etc. I have just frozen in front of them. Other than that I've only seen the ward registrar twice and had one interview with the nurses. This makes me feel there's no real attempt to find the root of my anxiety/depression.

Things go missing here, cigarettes, tapes, etc. Often patients take them, they can't help themselves.

[Did the respondent do anything?] We bring it up, but not a lot gets done about it.

These are selected comments and it should be emphasized that the positive ones are far more numerous. Nevertheless, they do illustrate that at least some respondents are able and willing to bring up criticisms, small or large, and show that even a single comment can sometimes speak volumes about life on the ward.

The impact of the process

What then, of my two original questions? As I warned, I do not have any unequivocal answers to them, but our experience does take us some way towards answers. It is easier to see progress in relation to the second question concerning the usefulness of the Critical Incident Technique. One major question that must be directed at any such method is whether it is capable of eliciting criticisms, because of the almost universal reluctance of respondents to express negative views about health services. As I hope the examples illustrate, the Critical Incident Technique certainly does pick up some negative messages. It is possible, then, for a user to articulate to an interviewer, during a relatively brief interview, quite deep dissatisfactions and misgivings, as well as responses which can make the alert reader sit up and ask whether something is seriously amiss in a particular area. (Interestingly, staff responses can sometimes provide perspectives from a complementary angle which can build up the picture with an extra dimension.)

More mundane criticisms are fairly frequent, of such things as the lack of constructive activity, the food, and – depending on very local circumstances – physical amenities, personal clothing, and the security of one's own belongings. Conversely, appreciation of constructive activity, and of trips outside the hospital, is warmly conveyed; as is appreciation of caring and attentive staff. This two-sided picture, incidentally, seems to me to be extremely important in conveying to staff that much can be done within existing constraints, and when it is done it really has an effect.

The Critical Incident Technique can, therefore, uncover much that is interesting and has the ring of truth. Sometimes individual responses corroborate each other, but the technique as we deploy it is not designed to provide systematic 'triangulation', so such corroboration is sporadic. There is, then, no independent validation; and no definite refutation of the possible charge that CIT only scratches the surface. However, after seeing the results of 1,500 interviews I am much more positively inclined to the technique than when I started. It seems to me, at the very least, to offer the ends of pieces of string poking out from the organizational tangle, ends which can be grasped, teased out and followed to see what further truths lie beneath. That depends, of course, on the alertness of the readers of the incident sheets, and on their motivation to pursue the clues they offer.

This relates to the second question: given that the whole process is initiated and orchestrated by management, is there any chance that the users' views can make a real impact? I can only report my own provisional impressions. I do not subscribe to the view that professionals are universally arrogant and uncaring and the managers are cold accounting machines eager to cut expenditure. Such views fly in the face of logic and experience. So I was not surprised to find concern at the negatives and pleasure at the positives among the Top Teams charged with digesting the users' reports, and an expressed determination to put the wrongs right.

There is of course more to it. We know enough about psychiatric services in general – and here I am not talking about the particular hospitals where I have worked – to be able to say that a different truth is experienced by many users. Professionals are not always caring, sensitive and respectful, and management is not always well-directed and determined. I offer an interpretation based on the commonplace notion that an organization is a society, and institutions especially powerful societies. People's behaviour patterns within organizations are conditioned not only by their private beliefs but by what they believe to be expectations of those around them. This means that existing patterns of activity and neglect, work procedures, social interactions and so on are exceedingly difficult to shift – even when the majority of the members of a group privately believe that change is needed.

In such a situation the effect of another voice, a voice carrying authority and legitimacy, can be powerful. It can offer the chance to generate debate and discussion, and give courage to some to express what they might have thought unwelcome or minority views. The Total Quality approach as I have described it provides, in fact, a platform for not one but two voices, the owners of which have always been in the theatre but never in the spotlight. One is the voice of grassroots staff; and the other, given pride of place, is that of the service user. What is particularly important is that the legitimacy of the users' voice is acknowledged by the whole process, and lent force by the authority of management and professionals behind the process.

On the basis of what I have seen I would not, yet, renounce all cynicism. Each exercise has a long way to go and perhaps, still, the odds are stacked against true culture change. But I am heartened by my subjective impressions; I am convinced that at least some members of the management teams have taken the messages of the users extremely seriously, and that the intention is there to pursue constructive change. More than that it is impossible to say.

5 Consumers and the QUARTZ system

Steve Pilling

QUARTZ is a comprehensive quality assurance system for mental health services, particularly those providing continuing care. It has a potential application across a range of care groups beyond mental health. QUARTZ was developed at Research and Development for Psychiatry (RDP) by Rob Leiper, Paul Clifford, Tony Lavender and Stephen Pilling (Clifford *et al*, 1989). It has been piloted in a wide range of mental health services across four health districts and one local authority area. This chapter concentrates on the experience of user involvement gained in the pilot phase. The system has been subject to an extensive evaluation which is reported elsewhere (Hill and Leiper, 1992) and to which interested readers may refer. The system is currently being implemented in a wide range of statutory and voluntary agencies.

QUARTZ is a process orientated system of quality assurance and is fully described by Clifford *et al* (1989) and Leiper *et al* (1992a;b;c). However, the basic structure of the system is described below to provide a context for the discussion of user involvement. The development of QUARTZ began with two questions:

What characterizes quality services?

Quality services can be said to have a clear conception of the task, appropriate selection and delivery of the care provided, pay attention to users' quality of life, demonstrate good team functioning and show clear evidence of integration of the service within an overall care system. It is not difficult to find agreement on these characteristics of good quality services. Unfortunately it is just as easy to identify services where these characteristics are absent in part or whole. This leads to the second question:

If it is a straightforward matter to gain agreement on what constitutes quality services, why can it be so difficult to provide them?

There are a number of factors which contribute to the difficulty in providing quality services. They include poor quality staff or training, lack of management direction, poor clinical management systems, lack of awareness or knowledge of appropriate clinical functions, poor team functioning, and lack of involvement of users and carers. Again, it is not difficult to add to the list or gain agreement on it, but it is difficult to identify the precise contribution of each of these factors; there is obviously a complex interaction. In the development of the QUARTZ system it therefore seemed essential that the system acknowledge this complexity. It was decided that a primarily process orientated methodology would be better able to reflect this complexity than one which concentrated on outcome. Being aware of the overall context of the service is as important as reviewing every element of the service (a practical impossibility in most cases). For example, to promote user involvement as part of a quality initiative whilst not acknowledging or addressing its interaction with other aspects of the system is likely to lead to disappointment.

A review of the existing systems for audit and quality assurance (Clifford *et al*, 1989) identified a number of factors which are central to any effective audit or quality assurance system. These include:

1) An element of both internal and external review is necessary. Internal review is the process by which direct care staff, responsible for providing the care, are also involved in evaluating its quality and its outcome. However, to rely solely on methods of internal review can, and often does, lead to the avoidance of difficulties, concentration on internal matters and a lack of attention to the wider service system. To require an element of external review (that is the involvement of agencies with no direct responsibilities for the work of the service) is not to promote an inspectorial model, but rather to insist that the relationship to the wider system, including service user groups, carers groups and other agencies, is carefully considered.

2) The active involvement of users, clinicians/carers and management must be sought. If systems are to be successful they need to engage and promote ownership of the system by users, direct carers and clinical staff. However, without the support of management, a system is likely to be of little value. The interests of all these groups (which of course could be broadly the same) must be considered if the system is to have credibility and destructive clinician-manager or user-clinician splits are to be avoided.

3) The system should be an objective setting-based system which acknowledges the multi-faceted nature of the service provided. Objectivity

can be provided through appropriate information collection systems and the promotion of realistic and specific goals. Settings (i.e. wards, community teams, group homes) are the proper focus for quality assurance rather than professional groups. Of course, such settings may be multi-disciplinary, uni-disciplinary or multi-agency. The need to consider comprehensively the service provided means acknowledging and promoting the involvement of users and carers as well as external agencies with a legitimate interest in the care provided.

The components of the QUARTZ system

The QUARTZ system has two key components:

1. Quality Review Team (or Person/s)

QUARTZ can be implemented either by using a Quality Review Team (QRT), by an individual or by a looser collection of individuals than the QRT system described below. (A full description of the implementation methodology is given in Leiper *et al* (1992a)). As the pilot districts referred to above all operated with QRTs this method will be described here. QRTs in the pilot districts were composed of a group of senior staff drawn from the services under review. (However, it should be noted that in some districts where QUARTZ is currently being implemented, service users are being trained as QRT members.) It is important that this group is representative, but it is equally important that the group is not narrowly defined so that it is comprised entirely of service or professional managers. Personal credibility with direct care staff and users, and the skill needed to do the job are crucial. The QRT is not an inspectorial group nor is it a managerial group; it stands to the side of the management system. Its relationship to the managerial and clinical structures can be mediated through a Quality Steering Group whose membership is drawn from those agencies under review. To give an example from one pilot district, the QRT consisted of: a psychologist, a consultant psychiatrist, two social workers (one from the hospital team, one from a locality team that manages a community care facility), the co-ordinator of a local voluntary group, a senior housing worker from one of the group homes in the district, the CPN team leader, a manager of one of the mental health centres and the unit's professional advisor for nursing.

2. The schedules

The QRT member is responsible for facilitating a setting's quality review. The process of a review is guided by a series of schedules and an

Table 1
The QUARTZ Schedules

Service resources

1.1 Staffing Resources
- A Composition of Staff
- B Staffing Levels
- C Staff Retention

1.2 Financial Resources
- A Budget – Information/Procedures
- B Budget – Structure/Adequacy

1.3 Environmental Quality
- A External Features
- B Client Facilities
- C Therapy/Work Facilities
- D Staff Facilities
- E Overall Internal Environment
- F Personal Security and Safety

Working practices

3.1 Policy and Procedures
- A ServiceAims
- B Referral/Selection/Admission
- C Programme Planning
- D Case Co-ordination
- E Service Review

3.2 Team Work
- A Team Functioning
- B Meeting Structure
- D Team Working
- E Leadership/Co-ordination

3.3 Users' Lives
- A Regulation of Client Activity
- G Leisure Use Skills
- B Staff/Client Relationships

External links

2.1 Community Links
- A Acceptance by Community
- B Integration with Community
- C Participation by Community

2.2 Agency Links
- A Significance of Links
- B Communication/Coordination

2.3 Relations with Management
- A Perceptions of Management
- B Management Structure
- C Functional Relationship with Management
- D Management's Views

2.4 Professional Support
- A Supportive Relationships
- B Training

Service provision

4.1 Service Utilization
- A Information Systems
- B Service Usage
- C Service Information Profile

4.2 Service Programme
- A Crisis Stabilization
- C Meeting Functioning
- B Advocacy
- C Personal Care Skills
- D Domestic Skills
- E Social/Relationship Skills
- F Community Functioning Skills
- H Vocational/Work Skills
- I Educational Skills
- J Challenging Behaviours
- K Health Care
- L Mental Health – Medication
- M Mental Health– Psychological
- N Mental Health – Substance Abuse
- O External Resources and Supports

4.3 Individual Care
- A Individual Case Review
- B Case Work

4.4 Users' Views
- A User Consultation
- B User Feedback

accompanying manual (Leiper *et al*, (1992a;b;c.)). The schedules are grouped under four categories and are listed in Table 1.

As can be seen from the above table, there are a total of 14 schedules. The majority of the schedules relate directly to the services provided to users. One schedule, '4.4 Users' Views' is specifically concerned with the views of users and will be described in some detail. The schedule has two parts. Part A (User Consultation) is essentially an audit of a setting's methods and motives for user involvement and consultation. Its purpose is to help a setting understand what has been gained from user involvement. For some settings this may reveal serious gaps in their systems for consultation and problems with staff attitudes where work is needed, for others it may mean the refinement and enhancement of existing systems. Part B (User Feedback) is concerned with actual methods of user consultation employed by the setting and is the least prescriptive of all the QUARTZ schedules. It describes and advises on the use of a number of approaches including: questionnaire based surveys, individual interviews, group meetings, the use of advocacy services and links with existing user representative groups (e.g. Patients Councils); all of which may be used to facilitate the collection of user views.

It is not intended that all the schedules be used in a single review. Typically, four to seven will be selected following an initial discussion between the reviewer and the staff team. This selection may or may not include 'Users' Views' but the majority of the services in the pilot study chose to include it. Other services may choose to make the requirement to address the issue of user involvement clear. For example, a mental health service currently implementing the system has decided that all reviews must use the 'Users' Views' schedule.

The purpose of the schedules is to provide a comprehensive quality review to a setting through the provision of a structure to examine all aspects of a setting's work. Whatever schedules are used, all information collected is fed back to the staff team highlighting both the strengths and weaknesses of the service. Following the feedback of this information the final stage of the review is a goal setting exercise, in which the setting's staff meet with the reviewer and generate a list of action goals aimed at improving and maintaining service quality. The feedback generated from the schedules and action goals form the basis of the setting's quality report. Invariably dates are attached to goals and a cyclical process of review is thereby established.

As can be seen from the above description the QUARTZ system is primarily a staff based system of quality assurance. The rationale for this has not developed from tradition, ignorance or contempt for users' views. It is based on the belief that in virtually all services staff are the primary determinants of the quality of care provided and therefore need to be at the centre of any QA system if there is to be lasting positive change. However, the system cannot work if it is dependent solely on the staff group; a culture has to be established which values and promotes the development of quality. This is primarily the responsibility of management, but users can and should be involved in the promotion and development of that culture.

Involving users in QUARTZ

There are two primary methods by which users can be involved. The first, already described above, is through the direct feedback of their views by participation in the completion of the 'Users' Views' schedule. The second is concerned with the developmental and facilitative role that users can play. This can take a number of forms with regard to QUARTZ. It includes providing advocates for users who need assistance to participate in the feedback process. Alternatively, users may facilitate the establishment of a forum for the obtaining of users' views. Users or user groups may be represented on Steering Groups charged with the implementation of a QUARTZ system. Finally, users may be involved as reviewers through membership of a QRT.

QUARTZ continues to develop and enhance its methods of user involvement. The broad structures and possibilities for involvement have been set out above. Something of the experience of engaging users in the process may be obtained from the four examples given below. These examples are not selected because of their representativeness or their high quality; they were chosen simply as the last four reviews completed by a QRT (in a pilot district) of which the author was a member. They show therefore something of the strengths and weaknesses of QUARTZ as a means of developing user involvement in monitoring services.

1. A psychiatric day hospital

This 40 place unit had a well established staff group and was generally regarded as good service within the wider district services. The reviewer, who had good contacts with local user groups, had completed a number of schedules with the staff before approaching the Patients' Council in the Day Hospital. The reviewer felt that a number of important issues had arisen in the course of the review work with the staff that required user comment and involvement. Then there was a discussion with the Council of the issues so far identified, and to these were added issues raised by the Council. There followed considerable discussion of the most effective way to obtain the views of a large patient group (fifty plus), many of whom did not attend the Patients' Council. Eventually it was decided to develop a brief (15 item) questionnaire for distribution to all

48

patients. Further discussion then ensued with regard to the responsibility for the distribution of the questionnaire; it was impractical for the reviewer and both staff and Patients' Council felt their roles may be compromised by getting involved in the distribution of the questionnaire. Eventually, with the help of a few members of the Council, the issue was resolved and the questionnaires distributed. (A total of 25 responses were received to the 50 questionnaires sent out.)

A number of issues emerged from the survey that were to find their way into the final quality report. The first concerned the lack of privacy within the unit for day patients, the second focused on the need for specific advice on welfare rights; and the third concerned the need for the Patients' Council to develop better links with the local Users' Forum. Interestingly, the day hospital staff had been convinced that patients received a very poor service from their general practitioners, a view they were sure that the patients would share. The survey revealed widespread satisfaction with GPs, a result which, despite the difficulty in interpreting the results of such surveys, leads to further re-examination of the unit's relationship with GPs. In addition to the clear goals identified, the process of user involvement and consultation seems to have had a positive impact on the whole service.

2. Staffed group home (I)

This was a much smaller setting than the day hospital and so a very different method of consultation was chosen. Again, the initial stage consisted of the completion of a number of schedules with the staff group. This proved useful for both staff and reviewer in thinking about the issues that it would be particularly important to discuss with users. The users were informed about progress with the review and then were asked about how they wished to be involved. All wanted to be interviewed about the project in order to discuss with the reviewer the questions that had arisen in the discussion with the staff, as well as their own concerns. Three people chose to meet with the reviewer as a group; the remaining four people wanted to be interviewed individually. A number of specific concerns emerged from the user interviews. Some, such as locks on bedroom doors and a house visitors' policy, had already been identified as part of the review and the discussion with users centred on clarification of the issues so that clear action plans could be developed which had the support of all involved. One issue not identified in discussion with staff centred on the lack of structured activity in the house. This desire for structured activity ran contrary to the staff view that it was desirable for most activity to take place outside the house. This led to the most useful outcome of the review because it pushed the staff and the residents into a discussion about policy that was needed but had not so far taken place.

Finally, the residents complained about the lack of information on and explanation of their illnesses and the treatment given by professionals outside the house. It was agreed that staff would assist the residents in obtaining this information by whatever means seemed appropriate.

3. Staffed group home (II)

In this six person group home, consultation with users followed a similar pattern to that of the group home described above with a mix of individual and group interviews. The project had been open for some time, the physical state of the building was deteriorating. There was considerable dissatisfaction with this expressed by the users which echoed a theme from the work with the staff. The review provided a useful context in which the views of both users and staff came together. It also strengthened the setting in its discussions with managers for increased resources. The major issue that emerged from the interviews with users centred on the staff's involvement in the house. The staff and management of the setting were very concerned to preserve and promote the setting as the home of the residents, and as a consequence, avoided any activity in the house other than was deemed to be absolutely necessary. For example, despite the presence of an office in the group home, all paperwork was done at the agency's head office. However, it emerged from the interviews that the residents liked having staff around and very much wanted the office to be used for paperwork etc. This lead to further discussions in the house about the nature of the relationship between staff and residents in a way which had not occurred before, despite regular meetings and a basically sound relationship between staff and residents.

4. A psychogeriatric day hospital

The final example chosen raises a number of interesting issues about user involvement. It was not a successful review as a final report was not produced. This was primarily due to major changes in management structure during the review of the setting. Four out of five of the senior managers responsible for the service changed posts during the time of the review and it was impossible to provide the continuity that is required for a successful review. Nevertheless the majority of the review was completed although the 'Users' Views' schedule was not. It might be assumed that this was the result of the cognitive state of the users of the service; for example, many could have been suffering from dementia and so would have had considerable problems in contributing effectively. However, an examination of the Service Utilization schedule showed this not to be the case. This, of course, raises an immediate concern about the possible stereotyping of older people and the lack of consultation is worrying from that point of view alone. However, it also raises an additional question; who are the users of this service? In a setting with the explicit goal of providing a respite service, should not carers and families be seen as users of services? This, of course, raises the question as to how much families and other carers are also users of other mental health services. The challenge for QUARTZ and other QA systems identified by this example is first, to develop systems that can engage users in some way, however severe the nature of their disability, and secondly to engage carers where appropriate in the reviewing of service quality.

As indicated earlier QUARTZ has been subject to a detailed evaluation which is reported elsewhere (Hill and Leiper, 1992). However, for the purposes of this chapter it may be helpful to report at the anecdotal level the views expressed by users of services on the QUARTZ system. In all the settings in the pilot phase there has been positive feedback from users. The general feeling reported was one of validation of their views and pleasure from involvement in the review of services which are designed to serve them. The staff also report valuing user involvement and in most cases it appeared to stimulate a fresh dialogue between users and staff.

Conclusion

QUARTZ is a comprehensive quality assurance system which addresses both directly and indirectly the services provided to users. It is primarily a staff based system but a number of schedules address users' concerns and user involvement. It is a process orientated approach and demands considerable management and staff commitment. In the pilot phase QUARTZ has been valued by the majority of staff and users who have been involved.

The examples given above show that the QUARTZ system is able to engage the concerns of users in a real and meaningful way. In all the cases described above, where the outcome was positive, it can be argued that the major contribution of the system has been to extend and develop a dialogue between staff and users. In doing so QUARTZ points to the key area in developing user involvement in services: the need for staff and users to talk to each other about the difficulties which they face in delivering and receiving mental health services. In an area where rhetoric and ideology often appear to reduce the delivery of mental health services to little more than a political power struggle it is important that any system which develops a dialogue beyond such a banal point is encouraged. By developing this dialogue as part of a wider review of the quality of services QUARTZ may help prevent the marginalization that has occurred in many projects which have seen user involvement in isolation as the primary means of improving service quality.

6 The Inside Quality Assurance programme

Leonie Kellaher and Maggie Veitch

The Caring in Homes Initiative was set up in 1989 to follow up some of the recommendations made by the Wagner Report, *Residential Care: a Positive Choice* (HMSO, 1988). Five programmes make up the Initiative, commissioned and funded by the Department of Health. Each is intended, by different approaches, to widen knowledge and understanding across the wide range of residential settings. The programmes within the Initiative are all concerned with the way settings work and how they can be reconsidered with different groups of people in mind. The boundaries of residential care as the Initiative defines them are rather fluid, so that both the traditional type of residential setting and the less traditional, such as small group living arrangements, are included.

The programme outlined here, Inside Quality Assurance, is about understanding, developing and changing life in residential settings from the inside, along lines suggested by the 'insiders': residents, staff and others who have experience of residential life. The programme aims to develop and test a system for Self Evaluation which will be available as an Action Pack by the middle of 1992. The objective is to develop a process which can be used by homes themselves in ways which residents, staff and others think are appropriate.

This paper identifies the building blocks as they have been developed so far. Ideas are still emerging as different groups adapt the process and find ways of working that suit them. For this reason it should be stressed that this is only an outline of what is covered in greater detail in the Action Pack. However, as well as describing the IQA process, attention is drawn here to some of the consequences to have come out of people's attempts at the IQA Self Evaluation.

The Centre for Environmental & Social Studies in Ageing (CESSA) at the Polytechnic of North London started the development of IQA with a number of basic ideas in mind. Many of these ideas appear in the Wagner Report; others arose out of our earlier work in residential homes for older

53

people (Willcocks, Peace and Kellaher, 1987). These are now being tested in homes for other groups such as children; people with physical impairments; people with learning difficulties; and those with, or recovering from, mental illness. The terminology we are using has shifted a little, but the interpretations and the process itself are very different from the kind of consumer study we were engaged in a decade ago.

One of the basic principles of self evaluation is the need to place the residents' interests centrally. Residents are, after all, the people who experience residential care intensively, even if only on occasions and for short periods. This does not mean, however, that the interests of others are put aside. One must acknowledge that in residential settings there are at least two sets of interests that are often at odds with each other: the residents' interests and the organization's interests. We are aiming here to put the residents absolutely centrally. However there are other people who we are taking into account in this: staff are almost as important as the residents; and then there are friends, relatives and other people who cross the residential threshold. The need to take account of the collective group is essential, since it constitutes the environment which, sometimes exclusively, surrounds and supports the individual resident. IQA Self Evaluation takes the view that the establishment should be a collectivity which allows individuals to be themselves. There is, however, a constant tension between the needs of the individual and those of the collective. IQA is one way of ensuring that the interests of the individual are not overlooked. IQA aims to give maximum significance to individual comment whilst considering ways of applying what they are saying to the collective. The practice of making individual care plans in some establishments is, or course, another approach to improving the quality of residents' lives, and there are areas of overlap between care planning for individuals and the collective IQA process which CESSA is developing.

It is increasingly being said that better listening is one of the keys to quality assurance in care provision. An important starting point was knowledge that many residents, albeit in a low-key way, can indicate residential preferences. The problems arise when there is no legitimate place for these expressions to be heard and then acted on. IQA is one way of opening a niche in organizational and administrative practice which can legitimately and systematically take account of the ordinary things which everyone thinks, and may want to say, about the settings in which they live.

From the start we wanted to develop a process which would take into serious account the voice of residents and staff. We believe that some information from 'insiders', no matter how incomplete, is better than none. We would want to get information from as many insiders who can be drawn to respond, but even one comment can be taken account of. Having said this, we recognize that with some residents there will be communication problems, and that in certain instances it will be necessary to 'translate' what people are trying to say.

These are just some of the principles which underlie our efforts so far. In the course of developmental work, we have adapted and expanded our original assumptions in response to the comments of those who have tested the pack. This paper describes what has been achieved in the course of development work up to early summer, 1991. The final phase of development will be completed by spring 1992, after further work and consultation with users in more than a hundred residential establishments for all client groups.

Inside Quality Assurance – what is it about?

IQA is about Self Evaluation; that means the people who have the most experience of residential life describing, in an open and organized way, how things are in their home, and what ideas they may have for future plans and different approaches. It is about changing the residential culture so that residents and those around them become more free to comment on things that affect their day-to-day lives. It aims to establish a continuing self-evaluation process; to describe, to measure, and set standards. This process makes available, as appropriate, details of the achievements and the difficulties of life and work in homes.

The IQA approach to self-evaluation is characterized by a number of features which are the means applied to achieve these aims. The main principles are these:

- it builds on what is already established in the home, its present aims and objectives, the people who care about the home;

- it starts gradually, with a commitment to listen, because any information from insiders is better than no information;

- it takes account of what each individual wants to say about his or her residential experiences;

- it adapts the IQA plan to fit the home, and the demands, capacities, expectations and aspirations of the residents;

- it systematically collects descriptions of residential life and work, under an ordered set of headings. The IQA topics are: physical care; making choices; expressing feelings; the setting itself, as somewhere to live; how things run; and what the atmosphere is like;

55

- it finds out what aspects of the home could be different (rather than asking about 'satisfaction');
- it organizes the information gathered, in order to plan the future direction of the home;
- it shares thinking and comes to terms with differences as well as common ground;
- it is aware that offering support is necessary for residents, staff and others as they try out something different.

IQA – what does the whole process look like?

We are concerned to develop a process that will persist, that won't be a flash in the pan, that can have some roots. IQA is about establishing a *continuous* process of self-evaluation. This process over time is represented in Figure 1.

The ideal is improvement of quality, and there are several possible indicators of this. The Self Evaluation process endeavours to produce better planning in the home, resulting in increased choice for all concerned because

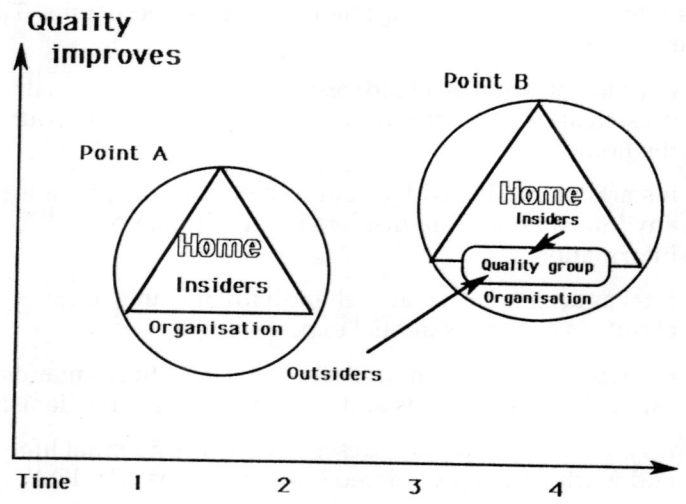

Figure 1 The IQA process over time

56

more views have been heard. In this way IQA can contribute to more equal opportunities for the residents. For example, the management of a home may previously (at point A) have been excessively biased in the direction of organization and administration, but at point B, once an ongoing IQA process has been established, a balance of needs may be achieved which is more receptive to individual requirements.

In IQA, the home, and the ways in which it may have habitually worked, becomes open to questioning (see Figure 2). This questioning does not have to be challenging or critical; indeed, in many instances it will be a positive and reinforcing process which indicates the areas in which the home is working well. The setting up of a Quality Group, as a first step in IQA, is the way in which new interests can be introduced. It is the main element and is intended to be the engine of this process. The quality group is made up of insiders and outsiders, and represents the home as a whole. What might happen between points A and B is that the outsiders become formally integrated or brought into the establishment and in that way, begin to break down barriers, and to do something to shift any tendencies to entrenched procedures. The Quality Group is crucial. It is responsible for setting in motion and completing the IQA process.

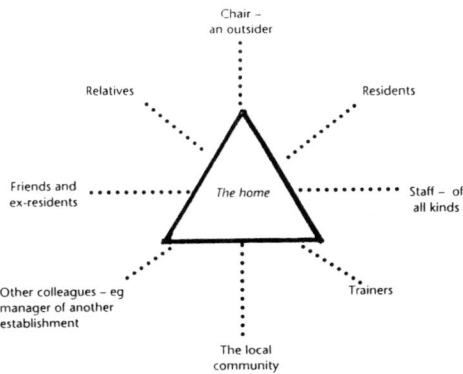

Figure 2   The IQA – Insiders and Outsiders

The 'insiders' will generally include the following groups of people: residents; the head of the home and the senior staff; staff whose roles cover day-to-day care and domestic duties within the home; and possible specialist staff. The 'outsiders', people who come into the home either regularly or occasionally, but who are in a position to make sensitive comments about the way things run, will include a much wider range of people: relatives and friends; field social workers; management committee members and trustees; home management staff who work for the agency, organization or authority which owns the home; GPs; community nurses; leagues of friends or supporters' groups. The list of possibilities is a long one and will be different for every home.

All these people have an interest in the home and the way it works. The IQA process depends upon the formation of a Quality Group, made up of people like this who, by combining the knowledge of insiders with the fresh perspective which outsiders can offer, can plan for the future in a sensitive and responsive way.

IQA – self evaluation: how?

The process of actually undertaking Self-Evaluation can be thought of as a sequence of stages. The first step is for the insiders and outsiders to meet as a Quality Group, representing everyone in the home. They establish:

a) the home's aims and strategies;

b) the aims and strategies of the self-evaluation;

c) roles and responsibilities of the group;

d) time limits for the evaluation.

The second, third and fourth steps cover the way in which information is collected about the establishment: both the residents and the staff are offered an individual 30-minute interview with one of the outsiders from the Quality Group (not the insiders) to collect information. Then others with an interest in the home, e.g. relatives, friends, and professionals, are asked to give their views by post.

The insiders are brought into play when, in Step 5, everyone's views are summarized anonymously on paper by the Quality Group under a series of main headings. Then in Step 6 information is sorted according to the category of interviewee and in a matrix of possibilities for action. This is a process of sorting under topic headings, scanning, and then making some preliminary decisions based on the various constituencies, about what is the weighting, what is the content, and how all this relates to a matrix concerned with action. The group considers: what can we do something about now; what can we never do anything about; what are we satisfied with; what do we think is working well; what can we put in our report as OK; what do we put in our report as needing attention. This matrix acts as a very rough guide to future plans. Step 7 is to provide provisional feedback to the whole group, to pool ideas, manage differences and check that the evaluation is on the right lines. Feedback is

Step 8: results are reported, conclusions drawn and plans for future action agreed. Finally, as Step 9, a written account is produced, summarizing individual views on each of the topics.

The Action Pack as it has so far been developed and tested is made up of a number of items which are intended to guide people to get started with IQA Self Evaluation themselves. The pack is intended to be adapted to meet the particular style and character of a home and the wishes of those taking part, especially the insiders. It contains:

- advice and suggestions for setting up a quality group and then for collecting, sorting and organizing information;

- topic sheets and prompt lists;

- guidance and scripts for using topic sheets;

- record sheets and sort sheets for organizing the information from the various groups.

It also includes:

- posters to illustrate the stages to be undertaken in IQA;

- prompt cards;

- a measure/scale to indicate degree of difference or change desired on particular topics.

Seven topics form the basis for getting people to describe their own experiences or observations in the interviews of Steps 2 and 3. These are: physical care; social care; emotional care; the place itself as somewhere to live; the physical environment; the way things are run; and the atmosphere – what does it feel like here. These topics are very broad in order to allow people to say something about every aspect of residential life. It is essential that people should be able to describe things as they experience them, not as a response to a checklist or questionnaire which represents someone else's view of how things might be. However, there is no reason why a home should not make up its own topic list. People are asked to describe how they feel about each of the set topic items, and then asked whether anything needs to be different. The same basic list is used for everyone, residents and staff alike.

The development of these topics took about a year, and continues. Our early trials showed no particular patterns, so we went back to something that was very general and covered all the facets of residential life. There are opportunities for residents, staff and others to introduce their particular perspective. We include in the pack a big plastic ruler marked one to nine with a sliding pointer. Some client groups are very happy to use this, other clients groups are really not – elderly residents for instance are uneasy with numbers and this particular scale. However, it allows the possibility of ascribing some numerical weight as to whether a situation needs to be 'a lot' different or 'hardly at all'. Residents are well able to describe their environment, and this applies even to older people who can often be reticent. In our earlier consumer study (Willcocks *et al*, 1987) we found very high rates of satisfaction with the environment reported which had little meaning. It was quite clear that many of the residents were simply not engaged with the questions. What may be happening in IQA is that the topics are open enough for people to begin to engage with them on their own terms and they are actually giving descriptions which are illuminating.

Improvement of quality: processes and outcomes

In seeking to facilitate change there are, inevitably, certain snags in the IQA system. Confidentiality, and the ability to attribute people's comments are extremely important issues. Nonetheless we believe that some of the benefits of the self-evaluation process can include: increased levels of awareness of aims and strategies; better relationships between people; increased confidence in individuals; a shared understanding and appreciation of collective living; an agenda for action and the possibility of change; better links with the local community and Inspection Units; and staff development may be more focused. This is in addition to the production of valuable information which can be put to various uses. This is probably a very ambitious list of what might emerge from the process. We aim for quite small, concrete changes but these can mean a great deal in environments which are often very static, if not entrenched. The slightest movement in these settings is really a very good sign. That is really what our programme is aiming to do.

7 Quality for people – Working in partnership

Alison Kerruish and Helen Smith

The Centre for Applied Psychology of Social Care (CAPSC) at the University of Kent has been funded to undertake a project in Bromley, Kent to develop ways of monitoring the quality of residential services for people with long-term mental health problems. The project is funded until the end of February 1993. This paper describes the progress in working with users to list the quality issues that concern them. Those issues can then be used by all participants in the service to bring about effective improvements.

The aim of the project is to support the development of high quality residential services by enabling users to comment on the services they receive. Residential services were chosen as the particular focus for a number of reasons. For this group of people the quality of service is very closely linked to their quality of life and it is therefore particularly important that they should have the opportunity to make their views known. Additionally, many of the people have just moved out of large institutions and are vulnerable as a result of years of disempowerment. Having spent twenty or thirty years in hospitals they may not know what to expect and may have nothing to compare the service with. This creates a challenge in finding out what people want out of the service when they have no knowledge of what the service might be expected to provide and no experience of high quality services.

Two other reasons for bothering to ask users about the quality of the service relate to the fundamentals of service provision. A year after the Rubber Windmill simulation of the internal market in the provision of health services, there was a review of progress. One of the reasons for the crash in the simulation was that users' and consumers' views were not taken into account and that is still the case, not just by those commissioning services but within the whole purchaser/provider framework (East Anglian RHA/Office of Public Management, 1990). An approach to the provision of mental health services based on the needs and wishes of service users will actually mean quite significant changes. Working with service users to develop a service profile and a plan for future development in one West Midlands district has meant significant changes. A SEARCH conference (Wertheimer, 1989) with equal numbers of workers and service users showed that the things that the mental health services have traditionally paid so much attention to – the treatments and therapy – were not what users valued and wanted. An approach based on people's needs could significantly shift the balance of provision.

Involving people who use services in defining quality issues and indicators could ensure that purchasers and providers are, in fact, aiming to provide something that is relevant and wanted by service users. This project aims to build on this natural resource of quality assurance experts. To date there have been very few **user-led** quality initiatives in services for people with mental health problems, especially in community-based settings, so it is hoped that the project will be an exiciting opportunity to strengthen the voice of those who use residential services.

The two major objectives of the project are:

- to enable residents to determine the components that make up a good quality service;

- to establish user-led methods for monitoring the quality of the service.

We are very clear that the collection of data is not an end in itself and that this research project is about collecting data as a prompt to action.

Most residents in the project will have moved to staffed housing in the Bromley area from Cane Hill hospital, a large Victorian institution in Coulsden, Surrey. Many will have spent years of their lives in the hospital, and as a consequence, will not know what to expect or what to compare it with. At the beginning of the project some had only just moved to the staffed houses and some had been living in the community for over a year. Bromley has an established Quality Assurance Monitoring Group, composed of professionals and users, which has a remit to comment on mental health services. Bromley also has a Mental Health Forum for carers and users, which has a remit to channel views on the service as well as training and finding advocates for people. They will both be an important part of the system of quality monitoring within which we are working.

Our overall aim, therefore, is to provide a feedback loop that will improve the quality of the service over time. It seemed important to think about the complexities of quality assurance and to acknowledge that one simple approach would not be adequate. The functions of quality assurance include:

- to ensure minimum standards are met;

- to enhance the quality of services over time;

- to provide coherent direction;
- to inform decisions about allocation of resources.

From this it is clear that there are certain things that policy makers have to do, some that purchasers have to do and some things that providers must do. A good quality assurance programme is one that co-ordinates a range of activities around it. Measures that access users' views fit into a number of these areas and encompass a range of different methods: monitoring through quality action groups, which in our definition have users and staff meeting together; consumer satisfaction surveys; advocacy; conscience register, (as used by British Airways). The conscience register is an anonymous reporting procedure which is concerned to measure the extent of a particular problem (eg pilots falling asleep on transatlantic flights) rather than to identify and blame individual people. This procedure, which is similar to Critical Incident Technique, could be adapted to mental health services so that staff and users could report or comment on incidents in an anonymous way. The point of quality assurance is to see how healthy the system is, not to find staff to blame. Complaints procedures are one obvious way of getting user feedback, but involving people in the planning and management of services provides that perspective before it is too late. At the purchaser level there is a need to administer consumer satisfaction surveys independently of providers and to involve users in the writing of community care plans to ensure that the service specification is consistent with the people's needs. Experience from the United States seems to show that a good quality service is only achieved through a strong purchasing agency. If you think that contracts are a way of changing the service you need to know that they are relevant to users' perceptions of what they need. The example of the SEARCH conference shows that we should not be *(see #p 62)* complacent about our knowledge of what users want. It is important to reflect users' needs in the specifications that are written and then purchasers need to know that the specifications are being met.

The three phases of this project are: the development of a number of components which define good practice from the users' point of view, *3 phases* the development of methods for monitoring the components (monitoring mechanisms), and the development of structures for implementing *of project.* these methods.

Quality for people in practice

The pilot in one of the houses used group discussions to collect information on what residents think is important for a good residential service.

The group discussions were facilitated in such a way as to enable residents to take an active role in determining issues for the quality components. This reflects the notion of 'working in partnership' with residents in the research. The pilot showed how essential it was to get to know the residents in the house before moving on to the group discussions. This was to establish trust between the researcher and the residents and also to give people the opportunity to decide whether or not they wished to participate. Additionally it enabled staff and residents to have a clearer understanding of what the research is all about and was beneficial for establishing trust with the staff in the houses. After the group discussions some volunteers from the pilot house worked in a group, facilitated by a researcher, to summarize all the information in order to draw out the key quality issues under each of five components. These components outline what residents have said they need to make a good quality service:

1. Relationships;

2. Equality and Empowerment;

3. Choice and Control;

4. Developing Skills;

5. Community Integration.

The quality component framework gives details and the staff actions, physical environment, information requirements, rights and responsibilities involved in each of the particular components. The equality and empowerment component, for example, covers staff/resident interaction, attention to physical health, the image the service projects to the outside world, involvement in care plans and citizenship rights. All components are expressed in terms of what residents need from the service.

In addition to the information on what residents view as important to them as receivers of services we need also to know what those working in, managing and commissioning services need to know about each service in order to ensure that it is meeting residents' needs. We are, therefore, developing simple but hopefully accurate ways of feeding different bits of information from residents to the different parts of the service system. The complexity of a housing service means that the quality of the service cannot be encapsulated in one method, but that many different types of methods are necessary to reflect the range of services and agencies involved. A number of feedback systems need to be established therefore, so that information about the service is coming from and going to many different sources. That information must be targeted at the group that can properly act upon it. The major agencies/ groups involved in the services – the commissioners, the providers, the house managers and the staff working in the houses all need to know different things about the service from the residents; but the sort of information people require should cover:

- day to day issues;
- specific views from residents about what is happening in the houses;
- inter-house issues;
- general information about what is happening in the houses;
- how active the service is in helping people live ordinary lives;
- issues that have funding implications;
- complaints.

Kinds of info. to be fed back to; service commisioners; providers; house managers; house staff.

One of the intentions of the project is to set up a number of ways of monitoring the quality of the residential service being offered to people. Five ways were identified and developed, which are currently in various stages of implementation:

- links to a resident's Individual Service Review;
- links to the Service's Operational or Facility Review;
- links with the Service's Residents' Association;
- an anonymous questionnaire, completed with help from an independent person, if required;
- a House Users Group, facilitated by an independent person.

5 ways of Monitoring quality

The lessons so far from the project are that service users in residential settings are very able and willing to give their views. The information people gave in the group discussions was enormous both in quantity and quality. Deriving a quality component framework from all the information was made easy by virtue of the range of issues and variety of topics that people raised, and was only complicated by the sheer volume of information that people had given. The residents are, on the whole, very eager to take part in questionnaires, House User Groups and the Residents' Association. The toughest challenge of the project is now in working with the service to implement these initiatives and to ensure that the service responds to what its residents have to say about it.

We would like to acknowledge the help of Christine Reardon for her contribution to the ideas presented in this paper.

8 Power, change and mediation as issues in Quality Assurance

Richard Grover

> Life depends on the polarity between activity and receptivity. This maintains tension, every adjustment of which manifests itself as a change, a process in life. If this state of tension, this potential, were to cease, there would no longer be a criterion for life – life could no longer express itself. On the other hand, these polar oppositions, these tensions, are constantly being generated anew by the changes inherent in life. (I Ching,1951)

Tension is normally seen as something to be got rid of or avoided as something damaging to health. Yet it is essential to life for without it there would be no movement. Nothing would happen. How can this apparent paradox be resolved?

We have lost or we ignore the creative potential in tension. The world tends to be viewed in dualistic terms, of having to choose one side or the other, to see one as good/right and the other as bad/wrong. Within mental health services, where the fear of loss of control is commonplace, the failure to find productive ways of using the inherent tensions often leads to damaging outcomes. Users and staff come to view each other with increasing suspicion and fear, leading to caring objectives being translated into skirmishing and outright hostility. We need to look at the creative possibilities inherent in these tensions. In so looking we will find a potentially important role for systems of quality assurance.

Power

Tension is the energy that exists between polarities. Polarities are sources of power. The distribution and use of power is a matter of constant human concern with one party seeking to assert primacy over another. If the process is not to lead to schism then some accommodation of

67

differing views has to be arrived at, with each party deciding what it will give away in order to achieve something of what it wants. How much is given away and what a party can insist upon depends largely upon how power is distributed. Sometimes the balance is so uneven that one party becomes dominant and can insist on matters being resolved entirely upon terms that it defines.

Possessing a 'controlling interest' in power gives a group (most often a minority) the authority to specify certain required patterns of behaviour. It may be claimed that their exercise of that power is in the best interests of those with less power on the premise that they are ill, ignorant or inferior; the language becoming increasingly abusive as the powerful lose sympathy for those in their control. The capacity to act against the holders of power may be very limited and change may seem unlikely. But there will be an ever present tendency towards redressing the imbalance in power, even if this takes a long time in personal or group history and even if it leads to the loss of some things in the status quo that were considered beneficial.

Within social welfare provision there is a substantial imbalance of power between the helper and the helped. The imbalance is in the very nature of the relationship and is difficult to remove. The authority, knowledge and control over resources possessed by helpers means that they have greater power in key areas than those they seek to help. It is implicit in the helpers' role. They must recognize that this is the logical consequence of the structure within which they work and that it has an impact upon those with whom they work.

In the social welfare field power largely rests within the framework of a series of inter-connected pyramids. At their heads sit national and local politicians, hospital consultants, directors of social services, chief probation officers and so on. The bases of these pyramids have always been the client/customer/user/consumer, the greatest number with the least power.

At various times users have fought for, and occasionally been given, a greater say in the nature and delivery of services, although it is noticeable how little they have generally pushed for a say in service provision, no matter how modest. There is a battery of terms to describe this process: user involvement, user input, client choice, listening to users, users views, user empowerment etc.; the meanings having more to do with preconceptions and prejudice rather than clear statements of principle and practice. The term 'user empowerment' is to be preferred because ultimately we are talking about the distribution of power.

The various branches of social welfare incorporate the issue of empowerment in different ways. People who are deemed to be suffering a mental illness, for example, have a difficult time not just because of their illness but because of the response from both the public and the providers of services. Users may have to deal with hostility rooted in fear from both groups. Such negative influences are then reinforced through the adoption by service providers of the 'common sense' view that those who are in some way mentally ill are not capable of sharing decisions concerning the services they use. Their perceived illness disqualifies them from having their views and experiences taken into account since these will inevitably be seen as a reflection of the illness itself and thus lack the rationality that is thought to be essential to good judgment.

There are the beginnings of a recognition of the injustice inherent in such a view, and attempts to begin the redress the balance. But recent research carried out by MIND and the Roehampton Institute (MIND, 1991) confirms the picture of the majority of mental health service users believing that they are not consulted about the treatment given them and feeling others are making the major decisions affecting their lives. This sense of lack of control, and the consequent increased dependency upon others is then used to give credence to the view that people who suffer a mental illness have inherent limitations.

If mental health services are to effectively support the efforts made by people to regain their health and equilibrium, then recognition must be given to the disabling effect of loss of power and control in key areas of life. This includes not just the loss of control over factors within their everyday life, such as being made homeless or redundant, but also loss of control through their experiences of being in contact with the 'helping' services, experiences that give rise to what Ivan Illich has termed and documented as 'iatrogenic disease'. (Illich, 1977) This recognition must in turn lead to giving back to service users as much of the power that rests with the professionals and politicians as is manageable. The means whereby a resource is delivered can combine with the service content to enhance the self-esteem and sense of being in control that are crucial to the growth and maintenance of good health. This holds true so long as the service content is in itself likely to be beneficial to the users – an assumption that it is not always wise to make. When considering the content of a resource it should be remembered that what goes into a facility depends largely on the questions that are asked at the planning stage. In relation to this process it is as well to remember the observation that:

> There is no greater power than the right to define the question. From that right flows a set of necessary answers. If the service provider can effectively assert the right to define the appropriate question, he has the power to determine the need of his neighbour rather than meeting his neighbour's need. (McKnight, 1977)

If user empowerment is to be effectively developed then it must be capable of addressing the 'what' is to be delivered as well as the 'how' of delivery itself.

Change and mediation

Change is not an option in human affairs, it is an inevitability. The processes of change are constant and are a key to life. Without change there is stagnation, a staging post along the path to death. The apparent security gained from holding an unchanging position is an illusion. In facing change we are faced with a series of options. Change can be resisted, an ultimately hopeless task akin to commanding the waves to recede; it can be directed for the self-seeking purposes of a minority; or it can be embraced as the means whereby the greater well-being of a community can be enhanced. Change that is directed towards community betterment requires that the question of the location of power as it affects the nature and management of resources is addressed.

But change can generate fear; as if taking away what we know will reveal only insecurity and malevolent forces. Thus change that is forced through against the will of some members of a community will breed a resistance that may well undermine the original good intention.

How then is change to be mediated so that the polarities can work in greater harmony for the benefit of all? The key lies in the recognition of the commonality of interests, that everyone involved in a given situation can and needs to benefit from the changes that are to be brought about. Certain essential qualities in the process of mediating change therefore stand out:

- an absence of condemnation of any party;
- the finding of some common ground;
- the seeking of a means whereby views and experiences can be shared;
- action that is based upon the inherent interdependence of the parties concerned.

A role for quality assurance

Quality assurance, like user empowerment, is an emotive and often unclear term. Both ideas are now being given more serious attention as a result of receiving modest legislative backing. The White Paper (HMSO, 1989) refers to 'the quality of services', 'consulting users' and several other similar phrases. These terms are largely undefined, and probably intentionally so, as are the methods by which the requirements will be met. But a *requirement* there is and through pursuing this requirement much might be achieved.

So what is quality? Quality is a difficult concept since it would appear to be capable of referring to anything anyone chooses. A facility seen as providing a 'quality service' by one group may be thought lacking important facets by another. Within social welfare the quality of service can be defined by looking at the degree to which it achieves its stated aims and objectives. It can be argued that such a definition is no more than a postponement of the need to find a more substantial definition that tackles the issues of subjective experience. Such a working definition has one important advantage: it places the wider debate about quality in the context of considering the characteristics and objectives of particular elements of welfare services which can then involve all the parties concerned with that particular facility.

Quality assurance then logically becomes the process of matching practice to the stated aims and objectives, and assessing the shortfalls. But if it is truly an *assurance* programme then it must go further by proposing changes to practice to bring it in line with policy or, if necess- ary, changes to policy so that the facility better meets the needs of the users. If the programme is to be effective then there must also be a plan of action to bring about the agreed changes and the capacity to monitor their implementation and the outcome.

Change is thus an in-built and essential element to any programme of quality assurance. Here it differs from many other forms of organiza- tional intervention that may identify problems and may even insist that action is taken to remedy them, but which do not aid the process of bringing change about. Such an approach can provoke fear and lead to an even stronger resistance to change than previously existed. What is required is a facilitative intervention that recognizes the key role of providers and users in bringing about constructive change and which seeks to draw them together. Participants come to share an under- standing of the issues and recognize the advantage to themselves and others in resolving them. Once advantage is perceived then change can be positively sought after rather than blocked.

Social welfare provision is made up of a collection of stakeholders— people and groups who have a legitimate interest in particular facilities and action. However the focus of their interests will differ according to the nature of their particular stake. The challenge is to bring the differing interests together for the common purpose of maximizing the benefit to service users, the most significant, if least powerful stakeholders of all.

But what will be the consequence if quality assurance, and thus the process of change, is pursued without any direct reference being made to the users and with the providers doing it all? Firstly, such a process will be a reflection of the values and priorities of the service providers and funders alone. They may achieve the objectives they set themselves but if these are not shared by the users then they cannot be providing a quality service since they will not be meeting the needs of users. Secondly, such an approach to quality assurance ignores one of the basic issues of

71

power: to make judgments as to the quality of a facility without involving the users is tantamount to saying that their views (and by implication, they themselves) do not count for much. It ignores the gains to the individual in terms of an increased sense of self-worth that grows from having their views and feelings taken into account.

All the stakeholders in a service, users, purchasers, providers, the public and government, have some power but with users being the least powerful by far. In the great Victorian institutions the power of users may have been no more than the occasional ability to frustrate the intentions of their guardians. The same may be true in many contemporary settings. Redressing the imbalance in power should be seen as a prerequisite to more effective resources in all areas of mental health. Historically, substantial improvements in services have been born solely out of the concern of philanthropists and reformers. But now there is a new spirit at work that requires greater account to be taken of the direct experiences of users and their arising empowerment. What could past muster once as a good reform programme is no longer adequate.

Service providers must become able and willing to meet the growing, and healthy, aspirations of the user groups to be more involved in the services they use. The historic problem in pursuing this process has been long established prejudice and the lack of common ground upon which the discussion about the shifting of power could take place. A well structured quality assurance programme can provide that common ground, making it relatively safe to explore important areas in an ordered way and encouraging the removal of prejudice that grows only stronger when a group feels under attack.

Fear is the great inhibition to any possible settlement of the power issue. Fear of mental illness is endemic in society and extends to those who work in the mental health services. Those working in the systems can, by their utterances, significantly affect the wider public view. So if members of this group feel under threat as a result of power moving to the users then they have the capacity to undermine the process by raising alarm. The fear may be that the users will abuse their increasing power to the detriment of the providing staff, even to having power over them. Whatever rationality lies behind such a view there is also the fear that goes with losing entrenched power to others long held in some degree of subjugation. A parallel might be drawn with the struggle for women's rights as portrayed by Mary Wollstonecraft two hundred years ago: 'I do not wish them (women) to have power over men; but over themselves'. (Wollstonecraft, 1792)

We also need to be wary of imposing a false group identity on users and to remember that the majority are unlikely to be sufficiently assertive to effectively challenge the staff view. Far from keeping users at bay, the effort is to find an appropriate means by gaining their involvement in service planning and delivery. Such involvement will in itself be health giving because of the statement of being valued that is so made. Practical changes to services made in response to users' views will then further support the process of gaining autonomy and health. The movement of power to a representative group of users is a significant and essential step but it must not be confused with the need to empower each individual user. No-one, be it professional or fellow user, can replace the importance of direct experience of regaining some control over one's own life.

Effective quality assurance programmes need certain characteristics if they are to provide the meeting place for the different stakeholders, and the immediate service providers and users in particular. Given the institutional patterns of behaviour that can arise just as much in community based facilities as in old hospitals, substantive change is most likely to take place over many months rather than days. Both the staff and users need time to adjust to change and both will need to experience it so they might develop their faith in some new way of working. For users there will be a need to repeat the processes of involvement so that inhibitions, doubts and anxieties can be overcome through beneficial experience. If people's views have long been unsought, or if expressed, ignored, then they are right to be sceptical at any sudden burst of interest in their thoughts and wishes. A one-off programme of user involvement will prove ineffective. Continuing engagement is demanded that allows for the gradual building up of confidence and experience on all sides.

The process also has to be action orientated. There must be tangible benefits to as many of the participants as is possible. The users and immediate providers have to be involved in finding and implementing the solutions as well as identifying the problems. The power to act must therefore either reside in the staff and the users or, where that power lies further up the hierarchy, must be speedily used to support the decisions taken. Should these more distant, but powerful, stakeholders withhold their approval of the outcome of the quality assurance process then they will undermine not just the immediate decisions of the staff and users involved, but also the value to be gained from undertaking the process itself. Both staff and users will feel undervalued and unlikely to be willing to place any further effort in that direction.

Quality assurance programmes can thus mediate the movement of power between the stakeholders and support the process of change. Quality assurance cannot compel anything to happen. It works through consent and requires an initial commitment from those with the most power to see the traditional relationships change in pursuit of improvements in mental health resources.

One certainty is that new prophets and enthusiasms will arise to replace today's favourites and the energy given to developing and implementing quality assurance systems will wane. Even if such systems are found to be valuable tools the energy is likely to be drained out of them. Their creative application to service settings will give way to mechanical/institutional processes, where the objective will be to produce an acceptable report with as little disturbance as possible to the established routine. In any human service, and possibly never more so than in mental health, staff and managers are constantly facing situations that challenge their sense of order and security. There is then a strong wish to impose order, reducing the number of variables that have to be dealt with, and so reducing the stress upon themselves. Institutionalization (in the sense of unthinking repetition of behaviour approved of within the immediate social group) is a factor of the human condition and not of bricks and mortar.

Such tendencies must be seen as the rule in social welfare services generally and we should behave as if such restrictions on action and thinking are imminent. Although it is not possible to entirely eliminate the movement towards stagnation, steps can be taken to slow the pace and occasionally to bring about a reversal of the flow, instilling new energy into established processes. Within quality assurance programmes the distribution of power between the stakeholders presents an opportunity for maintaining energy. Ossification will be most pronounced where power rests overwhelmingly with one stakeholder. Where the power is more widely distributed it will be more difficult for a single stakeholder to settle into a restrictive pattern. The effective sharing of power between stakeholders, and particularly the staff and users can lead to a creative tension that may keep life flowing through the process year on year. 'Creative tension' is a phrase beloved of writers and policy makers who do not have to deal with the anger, hurt and disappointment that are present alongside the desired outcomes. But the crucial point remains that such expressions of energy are more desirable than monotony and stagnation because they contain within them the seeds of change and betterment.

The process is again a circular one. Quality assurance encourages the greater sharing of power. The sharing of power encourages the maintenance of an open process. The open system leads to a critical appraisal of the substantive issues. Such appraisals lead to beneficial change which in turn leads to further support for the sharing of power. The quality assurance programme provides the framework for action, but it must be a framework and not a prescription – a framework that is capable of adapting to constantly changing circumstances.

When things go well we speak of them having a rhythm. A good rhythm to the day ensures that things are well done. Rhythm does not exist in isolation, a thing that can be hooked out of the air. It is created by the interplay of the different forces at work, as in the wind creating ripples on the surface of the water. So it is in matters of social welfare. For there to be a true rhythm to the work the different forces (in this case, the stakeholders) have to be brought into some form of harmony with each other. If one totally overwhelms the others then a rhythm is not possible and sickness in various forms is the result. What we call quality assurance is in some respects nothing more than a means whereby attention can be given to finding a proper rhythm.

Section 2
PROBLEMS AND STRATEGIES IN CREATING CHANGE

9 The user perspective on mental health services: Its value and limitations

Dr Frank Holloway

Introduction

These are exciting times. Not since the brief flowering of the mental hygiene movement in the United States at the turn of the century has the voice of people with a mental illness been taken seriously. This chapter attempts to explore the value and limitations of the user perspective in the management and development of mental health services and in direct treatment and care.

The opinions of service users may have an effect on the services they receive in a number of ways. Firstly, users may communicate directly with service providers at the point of treatment or care. Although an open dialogue is critical to successful mental health practice, it can be particularly difficult to raise complaints or concerns within the relationship between the patient/client and the professional. Secondly, individual users may make formal complaints to management about the care that they have received. Analysis of complaints is of interest, but they represent only a fraction of the experiences of users. Thirdly, the views of users may be elicited by surveys, the results of which are then fed back to management and staff. Fourthly, user groups may provide direct feedback to management and become involved in the process of service development. Finally, users can actually run services (but this then puts them in the position of power over other service users, requiring similar structures of accountability to those in receipt of a service).

The chapter is written by a consultant psychiatrist with an interest in research and responsibility for managing a psychiatric service. The author is keenly aware of the humiliations that health and social services users and their families experience in their contact with 'caring' professionals. However the author is also convinced of the validity of the concept of mental illness, the effectiveness and importance of medication and other forms of treatment in relieving symptoms and the requirement (in certain circumstances) to admit people to hospital against their will and treat them compulsorily.

Why the interest in users' views of their care?

Health and social care professionals have always considered that their actions were being carried out in the best interests of their patients/ clients. However, concern over the quality of communication between the professional and service user and systematic assessment of users' actual views about the services that they receive are recent phenomena (Lebow, 1974; Gordon *et al*, 1979; Simpson *et al*, 1991). It is now widely accepted that knowledge of the user perspective will result in an improved system of health and social care (Kelman, 1976; Locker and Dunt, 1978).

Consumerism and the distrust of professionals

There has been a general trend to devalue the role of the 'professional' (with the possible exception of the accountancy profession!) which was particularly noticeable in the Thatcherite Britain of the 1980s. Professionals are accused of artificially creating an unjustified aura of expertise for reasons of self-interest. The principles and practices of biomedicine have been questioned and the historical development of the psychiatric profession has in particular undergone critical scrutiny (Scull, 1979; 1984).

This questioning approach to expertise has been paralleled by a rise in 'consumerism' (defined in the Concise Oxford English Dictionary as 'the protection of the interests of the purchasers of goods and services'). The Griffiths Report, which ushered in General Management to the National Health Service (NHS), explicitly enjoined the Management Board to ascertain the quality of the service delivered by seeking 'consumer' feedback (Jones *et al*, 1987). Following the implementation of the NHS White Paper 'Working for Patients' (HMSO, 1989a) purchasing authorities are including sampling of 'consumer' opinion in service contracts, and either carrying out the sampling themselves or requiring provider units to carry out the studies.

Concern that professionals (notably doctors) were distorting service priorities underlies the NHS and community care 'reforms' that have recently been introduced (HMSO, 1989a; 1989b; Pampling 1991). These have led to a separation between purchasing health and social services authorities and service providers. It is assumed that competition between providers will, within a 'mixed economy of care', lead to increased efficiency. Problems with this marketplace analogy will be discussed below.

'Antipsychiatry' and the patients' rights movement

The mental patients' rights movement, which originated in North America, has focused on the 'abuses that [users] suffered at the hands of a system that couldn't understand their particular life crises, but could only warehouse them and give them the seclusion room, the chemical straitjacket and other harsh treatment' (Brown, 1981). The movement owes much to radical politics, 'antipsychiatry', feminism and labelling theory. Tantam (1991) has commented on the skill of the 'antipsychiatrists' in using well-worn debating techniques such as guilt by association, their commitment to moral argument, their failure to distinguish statements of value from statements of fact and their capacity to induce anger amongst mainstream psychiatrists. The patients' rights movement shares these characteristics with 'antipsychiatry' and the increasingly influential perspective of normalization (Wolfensberger, 1972) or social role valorization (Wolfensberger, 1983).

The 'antipsychiatrists' won the public debate about mental illness in the late 1960s. Although the contemporary debate is more evenly divided, the patients' rights movement and normalization principles have undoubtedly had a significant influence on the stance of pressure groups such as MIND and the King's Fund. These bodies have in turn helped set the agenda for health and social service managers. One result of this influence has been an increasing interest in user empowerment and advocacy (Sang and O'Brien, 1984; Royal College of Psychiatrists, 1989; Anderson, 1989). Advocacy groups and patients' councils, largely funded by statutory services, are now flourishing throughout Britain. There is also general agreement that service users should be involved in planning and service development (Kingsley and Towell, 1988), although the impact of this involvement is yet to be clearly seen. User groups are publishing critiques of both local services and the wider service system (Camden Consortium, 1986; Lambeth MIND, 1988, Beeforth et al ,1990). There are even isolated examples of services that are run entirely by users (Chamberlin, 1988; Buckland, 1987).

From treatment compliance to collaboration

Health and social care professionals have very practical reasons to be concerned about the quality of their communication with their patients/clients (Simpson *et al*, 1991). There is evidence that compliance with treatment advice is more likely to occur where patients are satisfied with their care (Slater *et al*, 1982), whilst patient anxiety and dissatisfaction are related to lack of information, explanation and feedback from the doctor (Simpson *et al*, 1991). Failure of compliance with medication is a routine cause of relapse and readmission for patients who suffer from illnesses such as schizophrenia, severe depression and mania. The problem of treatment compliance receives surprisingly little attention in psychiatric practice (Van Putten, 1974). Recently this problem of ensuring compliance has been reformulated as a need to enhance collaboration between the user, carers and services (Corrigan *et al*, 1990).

It is also being increasingly recognized that effective psychiatric rehabilitation depends crucially on identifying rehabilitation goals that are
seen as both important and achievable by the service user (MacCarthy *et
al*, 1986). The significance of the often very sophisticated health beliefs
that people hold, both about medical problems in general (Armstrong, 1989)
and about mental health difficulties (Strauss and Estroff, 1989) is now
acknowledged. Detailed exploration of the frames of reference and coping
strategies of people who hear voices can lead to ideas about treatment that
challenge traditional psychiatric practices (Romme and Escher, 1989).

Consumer opinion and the process and outcome of care

Consumer opinion may serve as an index of the outcome of care or the
quality of the service that is provided (Findlay-Jones, 1983). Controlled
studies of alternatives to inpatient treatment that have involved long-
term community support have demonstrated increased satisfaction
amongst both patients and carers for community-based treatment (Stein
and Test, 1980; Fenton *et al*, 1979; Hoult *et al*, 1983). Evidence is also
accumulating that former long-stay hospital residents prefer the new
services (Pickard *et al*, 1992), despite significant concerns prior to leaving
the hospital (Abrahamson and Brenner, 1982; Abrahamson *et al*, 1989).
Qualitative studies of user views are a rich source of information on
users' priorities and problems (Lehman *et al*, 1982a; Kay and Legg, 1986;
Lieberman and Strauss, 1986; Holloway, 1989; Gregoire, 1990).

Users' opinions of service, can usefully be explored indirectly by
looking at the uptake of services. Bender and Pilling (1985) found that
people who dropped out from a verbally-oriented local authority day
centre were less intelligent and articulate than those who continued to
attend, the clear implication being that in fostering such a culture staff
were covertly excluding people with more severe psychiatric disabilities.
Studies of consumer opinion are often biased by failing to take account
of patients who drop out of the service, who are likely to be less satisfied
with their care than those who remain in contact.

There is much current interest in measuring the impact of mental
health services on the quality of life (QOL) of service users (Wilkinson *et
al*, 1991). Quality of life is an elusive concept, despite the enthusiasm with
which it is embraced by health economists. One influential QOL model
focuses on objective life conditions, subjective satisfaction in life domains
and the relationship between these and overall sense of well-being
(Lehman *et al*, 1982b; Lehman 1983). This literature produces interesting
indicators of the areas of concern in patients' lives which should be
addressed, although these issues are brought to life much more vividly
by investigating the verbatim responses of the patients than by the use
of rating scales and multi-variate statistics (Lehman *et al*, 1982a).

Yet another reason for exploring users' views of their care is to try to improve understanding of the process of care. It is often not clear in mental health services what aspects of the treatment and care that are provided are actually beneficial. Evaluative literature tends to adopt a 'black box' model of care. This has resulted in a shameful complacency about what actually goes on in care settings. One common theme to studies of users' experiences is the frequency of the complaint that services are poor at communicating with patients/clients (Locker and Dunt, 1978; Simpson *et al*, 1991). A more specific example is provided by the data on the attitudes of long-term day care users, which strongly suggests that day care plays a role very similar to that of paid work for people in employment (Holloway, 1989). If this analysis is accepted it follows that the prime focus of day care should be to emphasise healthy functioning.

Limitations of the user perspective

It has now been accepted albeit grudgingly by some professionals, that the user perspective on the delivery of health and social services is important (Kelman, 1976). However there are significant difficulties in accepting uncritically information or advice simply because it reflects, in some way or another, the opinion of service users.

The consumer analogy and mental health services

Much of the rhetoric behind the current interest in users views about services, and indeed the research that has been carried out in the field, is based on the model of the service user as a consumer. This model is unsatisfactory. Consumers purchase goods and services, which are sold (preferably in competition) in the market place. However consumers of health and social care are also 'work objects', submitting more or less willingly to the ministrations of the caring agencies (Stacey, 1976). Although by no means wholly passive actors in the receipt of care, the position of service user is profoundly different to the purchaser of cornflakes in the supermarket. Stacey (1976) has argued that the consumer model should be replaced by the concept of a partnership between patient/client and professional (albeit a very unequal one in terms of power and prestige). This partnership is very difficult to sustain, and there are many mechanisms in place to 'reduce patients to non-participating work objects' (Stacey, 1976). These mechanisms, in part, represent understandable psychological reactions by caring professionals to their emotionally very difficult tasks.

Service users have little or no choice about what is offered to them and are unlikely to be aware of the range of potential options available for dealing with their particular predicament. To be truly effective in judging the quality of the services that are provided, the 'consumer' would have to have an equivalent understanding of the nature of their problem and the likely outcome of the interventions that are offered to the average caring professional. This is clearly impossible. In reality the 'consumer' of services is often operating in a conceptual and informational vacuum.

The development of an internal market in health care in Britain threatens, ironically, further to reduce the choice of individual patients. The place that doctors held in the decision-making process will be taken by health authorities, which will become 'the people's advocates...act[ing] as discriminating purchasers by becoming expert in assessing health needs and monitoring the quality and effectiveness of health care' (Pampling, 1991). These authorities will seek information about users' views by carrying out surveys of consumer opinion, but the assessment of need will remain firmly within professional hands and at considerable remove from the point of care. Similar mechanisms will operate within the social care arena.

Consumer surveys: methodological issues

The literature on 'consumer' attitudes towards services is often of a poor scientific standard. There is in general a lack of clarity over the questions that the assessment of users' views can and should be addressing. These questions fall into three broad categories: measuring the quality of care; measuring the outcome of care; and identifying aspects of the service that require change (Locker and Dunt, 1978). Most studies that have been published are best seen as exploratory and hypothesis-generating rather than confirming or disconfirming hypotheses. On occasion the literature descends into anecdote. Anecdote can, of course, provide important insights into the workings of mental health services and the problems and priorities of users (and it provides useful fuel for flights of rhetoric). It is, however, a poor basis for policy development or the scientific understanding of complex phenomena.

Webb (Chapter 2) discusses in some detail the methodological difficulties that research in the field presents. In designing measures to assess attitudes it is important to be aware of such issues as response set (where the phrasing of the question constrains the answers provided), the desire of respondents to please the questioner and the level of 'no comment' responses (Lebow, 1974). There is a clear difficulty in obtaining responses from the most severely handicapped patients, and this has lead to their exclusion from surveys of attitudes to discharge from mental hospital (Abrahamson and Brenner, 1982). Obtaining representative samples is a major problem for surveys of 'consumer' opinion, and lack of data from service 'dropouts' artificially inflates reported satisfaction rates (Anderson, 1989).

84

Just asking people whether or not they are satisfied with their treatment is not particularly informative: people generally express an unrealistically high degree of satisfaction with the care that they receive (Lorefice and Borus, 1984; Slater *et al*, 1982). More revealing are questions that are designed to elicit comments about specific aspects of care. There is consequently a general trend in patient attitudes research towards a more focused approach (Fitzpatrick, 1991). However the fragmented nature of attitudes research has naturally led to the development of a plethora of measures, most of which have not been adequately assessed for their basic psychometric properties (reliability, validity and factor structure). One potentially useful way forward for researchers is to combine questions of specific relevance to a service with a broader measure of satisfaction, such as the Global Satisfaction Measure (Huxley and Mohamad, 1991).

Although most reported attitudes research is derived from self-report questionnaires and structured interviews (Jones *et al*, 1987), other methods are probably more effective in identifying the major concerns of users. Webb (Chapter 2) gives examples of the focus-group method, which is much used in the market-research industry and the application of card-sort techniques, which may be particularly effective where respondents are severely disabled by their illnesses. The rich vein of material that can be tapped by systematically analysing respondents' replies to open-ended questions has already been discussed.

Raising the scientific standard of the literature on users' perceptions of their care is a significant challenge. Attention by researchers (and funding agencies) to basic methodological issues would be a useful start. However further significant progress will depend on the development of a research tradition (ie people building upon others' work) and interdisciplinary cooperation in the research effort that includes both psychiatric professionals and social scientists. One important area for further research is the impact of ethnicity and culture on users' perceptions of their problems and experiences of the services. There is a need to develop a clearer research agenda that aims to link attitudes (of both staff and service users) with the process of care and its outcome. That this kind of research can be done was demonstrated over 20 years ago (see Wing and Brown, 1970).

Whose service is it anyway?

Although the focus of this chapter is on the views of the 'primary consumer' of mental health services it is important to recognise that we are all potential service users. Societal attitudes towards mental illness have a profound effect on people who become mentally ill (Bhugra, 1989). Studies of public opinion can identify the barriers that exist to people presenting for care with illnesses who would benefit from appropriate treatment. Public attitudes

85

towards the mentally ill also have an impact on service users' reintegration back into the community.

It is also important to acknowledge that mental health services have a significant function of social control. This is explicitly acknowledged within the 1983 Mental Health Act, which includes within the criteria for compulsory detention in hospital 'the protection of other persons': on occasion patients are detained in hospital not for their benefit but because they represent a significant risk to other people because of their mental illness.

The views of a consumer organization largely representing relatives, the National Schizophrenia Fellowship, are quite different from those of MIND, which very much takes on the role of advocate for the patient or client. Relatives' needs are legitimate and require separate consideration (MacCarthy, 1988). There is, in any case, a problem with the representativeness of existing consumer groups (Kelman, 1976). These groups contain a tiny minority of current and past service users. Although the voice of these groups appears authentic, they are clearly not representative of all consumers of services. At the least, the opinions and advice proffered must be subjected to the same critical analysis as the pronouncements of professional groups. We all have our axes to grind.

Traditionally medical practice has been primarily concerned with the individual patient at the point when they seek treatment. However in reality judgements have to be made about the allocation of scarce resources on the basis of the overall need for health care within a locality. The aspirations of individual service users must somehow be balanced against the needs of the community as a whole using a set of agreed and understood priorities. To put the issue crudely, a service solution that would be highly desirable for an individual service user may be inappropriate because its cost would deprive others in need of effective treatment or care.

Mental illness and the validity of users' judgements

Severe mental illnesses can significantly impair judgement, occasionally with disastrous consequences for the sufferer or their carers. Examples known to the author include a person who spent her life savings on unwanted gifts to casual aquaintances during a brief episode of mania (elevated mood), a depressed man who killed his wife because that was the only way to protect her from evil in the world and a man suffering from schizophrenia who sought advice on how he could remove his internal organs which he believed had been infiltrated by ball bearings. These examples have admittedly been chosen for their dramatic quality. More commonly the effects of severe mental illness are merely incapacitating for the sufferer and distressing for carers. Professionals are continually placed in the moral dilemma of either making decisions for their clients/patients and potentially acting in a coercive fashion or accepting potentially harmful decisions or behaviour that may be the result of the illness.

Most people who have severe disabilities as a consequence of their mental illnesses are perfectly able to comment on their circumstances (Holloway, 1989; Abrahamson et al, 1989; Pickard 1992). However their choices will be constrained by their experience. It was demonstrated over 20 years ago that the development of 'institutional' attitudes amongst long-stay psychiatric hospital residents (ie reluctance to consider leaving hospital) was associated with length of stay (patients who had been in hospital longer being less likely to want to leave) (Wing and Brown, 1970). Attitudes can, however, change. It has now been demonstrated that long-stay hospital residents, who initially tend to be reluctant to leave hospital, prefer life outside hospital (Pickard et al, 1992).

The issue of the validity of users' judgements about the quality of the services that they have received (that is the extent to which these opinions accurately reflect the quality of care actually provided) is in fact a general problem in the assessment of health care (Lebow, 1974). The major difficulty that service users face in accessing information about the problems that they are experiencing and the help that is potentially available has already been discussed. However, providing information is not a simple task. Professionals must enter into a dialogue with users and carers that takes seriously the views that they hold about mental illness. Health belief models are clearly both specific to individuals and culturally determined, and the theoretical and practical implications of these models are yet to be adequately appreciated.

Conclusion

This chapter has attempted to argue that systematic assessment of the opinions of service users, combined with a more collaborative relationship between professionals and their patients/clients and between the statutory services and user groups, would greatly benefit mental health services. However the user perspective, like all other viewpoints, is a partial one and must be subjected to the same critical scrutiny as the opinions of professionals, service managers and political decision-makers.

10 What does it mean to have user participation in planning?

Marion Beeforth

For user participation in the planning of mental health services to be successful, professionals will need to change their viewpoint. In the past, providers of mental health services have assumed that those in receipt of their services have no valid opinions about how they are treated. This traditional approach is characterized by the professional view that:

- we are providers of mental health services;
- we know what is best;
- we have to organize services;
- we must have user participation;
- let us set up a users' group;
- do we know any users we can ask?

A better model would be characterized by Figure 1. (see over)

Almost by definition their 'illness' has invalidated users' views about diagnosis, about treatment, about service delivery. That attitude is no longer widely acceptable and articles, conferences, books, policy documents are all calling for the views of users to be taken into account and user groups are beginning to have experience of getting involved in the planning process.

Experiences of user involvement in Brighton

In Brighton a strong user group called INSIGHT, which was set up in 1987 has achieved a great deal. INSIGHT aims to work for better mental health services both locally and nationally and their stated aims include the following points:

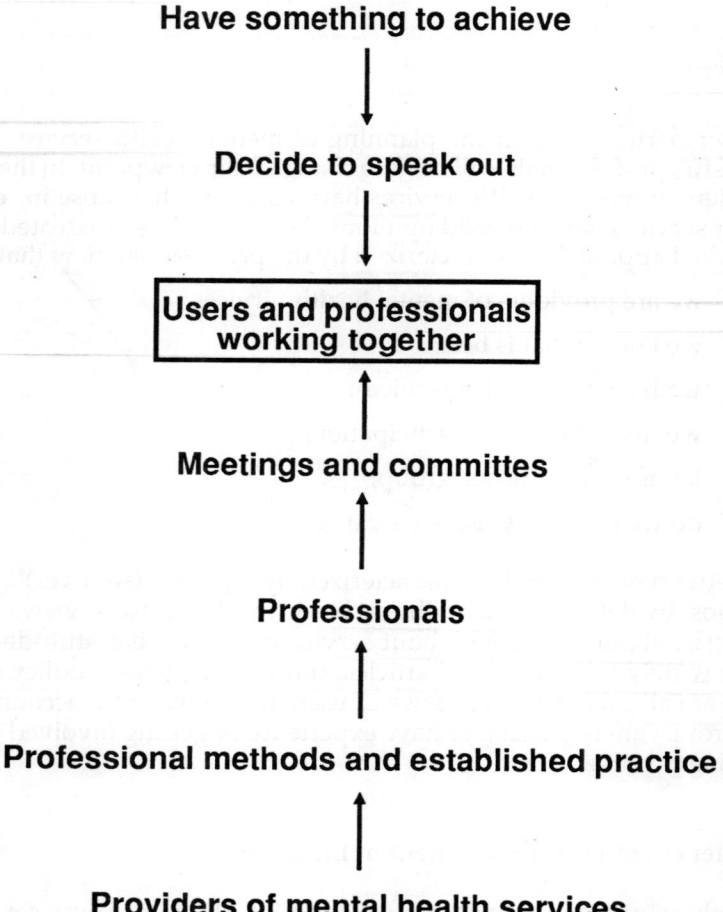

Users get together

Share their experiences

Have something to achieve

Decide to speak out

Users and professionals working together

Meetings and committes

Professionals

Professional methods and established practice

Providers of mental health services

Figure 1   User Participation model

We want to make it easier to get back to 'normal' life.

We want to eliminate the 'stigma' of mental illness.

We want very good community care.

We would like better housing, employment and understanding by the public.

Members of Brighton INSIGHT came together to share their experiences, to work together to try to change the way in which services are planned and delivered, to improve housing and job opportunities, and also to try to remove the stigma attached to mental health service users. We endeavour to work towards achieving our aims in a number of ways. We aim to make ourselves better informed by inviting speakers to our meetings; by sharing our experiences and ideas; and by speaking out with one voice because there is strength in numbers. One in four of our meetings are user only meetings and we have found that, at these meetings, users who do not normally have the confidence to speak at other meetings, do find themselves able to speak. Users can then gradually gain confidence to speak at other meetings. Our business meetings are not the most popular but they do give some training for onerous committee work. Members of Brighton INSIGHT have worked hard over the past five years to achieve their reputation, not only locally but also nationally.

On the face of it things are changing, but obviously user participation will not just happen, indeed it did not just happen in Brighton, it has to be made to work. One of the major questions is: 'Do workers actually want users to be involved?' or 'Are they already convinced that it will not work?' User involvement in the planning of mental health services means asking users to come on to providers' planning committees. It is important that the user representative is selected by users, rather than being invited as someone who professionals feel would 'fit in' with the committee. Professionals will have to learn to be prepared to accept a users' representative as an equal member of any committee and they should be prepared to listen to the users' points of view. It may well be difficult for professionals to do this and for them to take the representative seriously. As an example, are arrangements made to let users know when and if a meeting is cancelled? Are workers prepared to give them an opportunity to speak? Would you be prepared to offer them a lift? What makes the user viewpoint so relevant is the particular personal experience; but that same experience also makes the user vulnerable to personal attacks or patronizing attitudes from professionals. The counterbalance to the professionals' qualifications, training and assumed superiority is the strength which a user gains from sharing experiences with other users and coming to an understanding of how and why services fail. It is much harder to undermine the confidence of someone who is speaking from a collective viewpoint. For example, arguing for admission procedures to be changed so as to be more sensitive to distressed users, for example, has extra force when that argument is based in common experience.

The need for a strong user group

If users are to take a real role in the planning process then users, as a group, have to identify the issues about which they are most concerned. It is also necessary for users to consider whether it is worth taking the risk of speaking out. It is important to stress that it can be very daunting for users to speak out, but this becomes easier when user representatives are, at the same time, members of a strong user group. From this user group they will have the support and strength needed to do this difficult work. How would you feel being a member of a committee which might include your psychiatrist, as well as senior managers of a service you use?

There are also other issues in user involvement which are not yet so widely appreciated. Workers can further their careers and enhance their reputations because they pioneer 'user participation'. However, in many instances, this is achieved at the expense of the users themselves. It is true that the users' self esteem grows and they become more confident, but do their efforts gain them rewards in the form of well paid employment and better housing? Are the public more aware of their problems? Are mental health services any better? I am often asked to contribute comments and produce reports on mental health matters, but as I do not have a secretary, it seems to me that often I work harder than those professionals I meet on committees. I am committed to 'user participation' and I do enjoy the work; but is it right that in effect I 'pay' to do this work?

Also, the stress for users engaged in this work is considerable, the work is very demanding. If we did not have our mental health problems we would not be users; we are 'vulnerable' and we are often asked to do more than we feel able to. Yet this can be cited as evidence of the impossibility or rashness of user involvement. Workers stay in one post for two or three years on average before they move on. I have lived in the same area for more than twenty years and have seen generations of workers come and go. New workers arrive and they always want to start the process of user participation from scratch, regardless of the work that the local users have already achieved and those groups whose members are struggling to survive without support. Letting a user group be independent means giving enough support to allow the group to function without dictating to that group what it should, or should not, do. It is important for me to point out that if a

92

group is truly a user group then professionals should have no direct control over what happens after a group has been set up.

Sympathetic workers have been more than generous in sharing some of their skills with me; and individual workers have given their time freely to help me. However, not all users want to get involved and this should be accepted and respected. Some users have skills they acquired before they had problems but others have never had the opportunity to learn any such skills. Users need to have the resources to train and support those who want and need training. User groups do not properly fit into the same category as other voluntary organizations because they need to be resourced and supported in ways which have regard for users' particular needs.

Resources, support, training.

For full user involvement, users should be involved at all levels of decision making, not only in planning groups but in one to one therapeutic relationships and also in day and residential services. Can workers accept that some users may become workers and therefore also become colleagues; that some users may at some time actually make managerial decisions and that services may be user-run? This does not mean that the statutory agencies will then be absolved from providing resources and support for mental health services (thereby releasing funds for their other obligations eg children's services or services for elderly people). Are managers of mental health services really prepared to share control with users? As I have already said, mental health services are meant to benefit the user – but it does not always seem that this aim is achieved.

Involvement in the user participation movement is not easy. The work is demanding, we often find ourselves working alongside the same workers that we rely on to help us. However we are prepared to take the risks in order to get our message across.

How to involve users

Professionals often want to know how they can set up a new user group. It really does not happen quite like that. My suggestions for the various steps to be taken are as follows:

- get users together;
- leave them alone to talk;
- invite them onto committees;
- listen to what they say;
- give them information;
- pay their expenses.

93

User groups need to be able to publicize their existence and their work. New members can be contacted by word of mouth, from meeting members involved in advocacy or befriending services when they are working in hospitals and day centres. It would be very helpful if practitioners could see their way to recommending their patients/clients to go and see for themselves how the local groups work. The authorities can be disbelieving of the fact that users can speak up for themselves and think that they need someone else to represent their views. It is also often the case that, even if you have supported the setting up of a user group and helped in some way to persuade others that it is a good idea or have provided premises, nonetheless you may find yourself challenged by the users. You may find that your ideas do not always coincide with theirs. Again, even if your ideas are very much in line with theirs they may not want you to speak for them; they may prefer to speak for themselves but with your encouragement. Your help and support will always be welcome but you must allow the users to define how that support is to be used.

If the steps outlined above are followed you will have the basic necessities for a new user group. However, users are poor; they are usually on benefits; and they do not have access to typewriters, photocopiers, telephones, secretaries etc. The importance of the absence of these facilities is rarely appreciated by those who have grown accustomed to using them. It is amazing how much users can achieve with a fraction of the resources available to professionals. Working with user groups is a new way of working for providers of services! It can be a learning process for both users and professionals. Users' actual experiences can be more valuable than professionals' theory and practice.

Difficulties

There are many practical difficulties to be overcome. How do you avoid 'tokenism' – 'we have two users on our committee so that is all right?' Do you listen to the users? Do you take notice of what the users say? Not all users will have the skills necessary for this work, but accept that some do; and make it possible for the others to acquire these skills and accept also that we may need support. Users in Brighton are asked to attend a wide variety of meetings. These may include development meetings at which ideas are aired or specific project groups where issues such as rehabilitation, complaints procedure, advocacy etc are discussed. INSIGHT members sit on planning and steering groups, they have given valuable input to a peer advocacy scheme, they helped to establish a Brighton Users' Charter (before such charters became politically fashionable) and they are asked regularly to give talks and run training sessions.

The work that users do in the area of user participation can be very difficult for them. It is hard work. They need courage because their work is confrontational. They have to learn the 'jargon' and to be prepared to interrupt when they do not understand. Often users work more slowly than professionals. We have had our battles at meetings. I have already mentioned the problem of meetings being cancelled without notice. One INSIGHT member was told he was not fit to be a 'rep'. Why? Because he did not wear a tie, did not have a briefcase and arrived on his bicycle. I was once asked at a meeting: who wrote those notes for you? I can actually read and write! Professionals have to earn the trust of users.

We are not full time paid workers and this means that as well as lacking resources, as mentioned earlier, we are not necessarily going to be available when professional workers are. This is because we may well have jobs (however menial); or a family and a home to run. Everyone keeps telling us that we are vulnerable people, and we may well be using mental health services at the same time.

Making it work

It is important to remember that users do have rights and that both professionals and users have to learn how to make user participation work. Users would also like workers to accept that although we are users, we do have something of value to contribute and for workers to acknowledge that we will probably find it at least as stressful as the workers will. Workers have problems outside their working lives; and users have problems which are not secret. In the planning process both these types of problems have to be set aside, but it may be difficult for professionals to set aside their preformed perceptions of particular people. Do things always have to be done the way they are? Remember the suffragette movement and how hard they had to fight to get women the vote. Today it is universally accepted that women do have the right to vote. Why not put people first!

11 User views – From a provider's viewpoint

Sally Robbins

The involvement of users in service design and monitoring is a relatively new phenomenon. The introduction of this idea has coincided with a whole swathe of changes within the NHS which have been brought in by government action since the mid 1980s. I think it is true to say that all this has produced a radical shift in NHS culture and has altered the power balance in the organization beyond all recognition. The major change has been away from professional power and towards managerial and latterly towards 'consumer' power. Many professionals would probably concede, at least privately, that some of this power shift was necessary. However, there is a real debate about the extent to which the professionals should lose power.

Unease about the way this is perceived goes together with a recognition of professional power loss as a theme of this administration, common to education, local government, law and business as well as health. Sometimes it can feel as if there is an element of 'professional bashing' in all this, as if now the tables are turned and we are reaping the reward of (other) past abuse of professional power. To the well-meaning professional practitioner this can seem rather unfair, as well as rather scary. In fact the situation is further complicated by the way the NHS reforms work, giving power to GPs and Commissioners. Whilst they may be more in touch with users views than those who had power under the old dispensation, GPs and Commissioners are hardly the same as the actual service consumers. The introduction of user feedback systems needs to be considered against the background of threat, suspicion and doubt which all this engenders in the staff providing services.

Predictably, all this creates problems for those of us who are well-meaning but unsure about how best to involve service users in the management of service provision. Life would be much simpler if one were only sure of the way ahead, or else did not care. I feel a heavy responsibility to get my consultation with service users 'right', whilst recognizing that this is probably a contradiction in terms since the whole idea is to share power and hence responsibility. Linked to this is, of course, the simple fear that if I followed consumers, wishes I would make myself redundant. I recognize that my therapeutic relationships are rarely comfortable for those I work with, and I feel that this is often a necessary concomitant of personal growth and change. When those I work with do make substantial changes, many of them would not see this as connected with my work with them. In the main I do see the connection, but then to paraphrase the well know saying 'I would, wouldn't I'. If those I work with find the process difficult and uncomfortable and may not credit me with any part in the progress they make, how can I trust their judgment on how we run our service? The thorny question of who knows best arises from this quite easily. The difficulty of struggling with these thoughts and feelings is compounded by the speed of cultural change within the NHS. This has left many of us unsure of the level of sophistication which might be applied to the inclusion of users' views by those who manage us and those who now commission services.

The use of opinions and comments from service users in the management of service delivery raises three main questions for service providers:

- the cost and cost-effectiveness of eliciting meaningful user feedback;

- the problem of getting feedback information to the right people in our organization and then acting on it appropriately.;

- the question of how one develops services and how much the direction of developments is to be dictated by user opinion.

Eliciting feedback

There is a real dilemma for service providers who attempt to incorporate users' views into their self-monitoring processes. Essentially, the choice is between investing considerable time, money, and corporate effort in obtaining useful and reasonably accurate information or alternatively using these same resources for more immediate priorities in service delivery. There is a great temptation to do the latter whilst paying lip service to the former – recognizable as either the 'coming soon' or the 'quick and dirty' response to these issues. Either we dither about how best to incorporate consumer feedback into our service management; or we use a simple method of feedback, (preferably one which we can distort the results of) and present ourselves as being in touch with user's views.

Decisions about what to do about eliciting and using consumer views are further complicated by difficulties with the methodology of consumer feedback. The unreliable nature and poor validity of many survey methods has been well documented. (Lebow 1982, Webb, Chapter 2). Consumers only rarely make adverse comments and great care must be taken to maximize the chances of getting criticisms and suggestions which are representative of those receiving services. In service terms, of course, 'great care' translates as 'not quick or cheap'. This leaves the provider both unsure how much to trust any data which is forthcoming on the service, and needing to make hard choices about how much to spend on eliciting the information. In many ways the 'coming soon' position, in which we postpone the introduction of user feedback perhaps because we are unsure of how best to approach it and fearful of doing it inadequately, is quite attractive, especially to a busy harassed manager.

One example of the sort of situation which might make us wary of the accuracy of the answers we get when we attempt to consult those who use our services, has occurred several times in my own clinical work. It raises concerns about giving too much weight to the opinions we elicit. 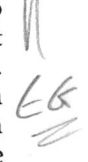 My work has mainly been with elderly people with mental health problems. Traditionally, hospital wards for such people have often been locked, although staff have had no legal right to forcibly detain those housed there. In trying to improve services, one obvious area for action is to put this situation right. Most of the elderly people themselves are not able to give a direct and consistent opinion on the matter, and they have great difficulty in articulating their opinions. Because of this, staff tend to rely on relatives, friends and carers to give a consumer view. When consulted many of these people actually want the doors to remain locked, whatever the legality of the situation or the experience of the elderly person. They say that the patients must be safeguarded from wandering out and getting lost and that this is of paramount importance. If you listen a little closer you hear some people whose pain about the condition of their friend or relative is too great for them to even contemplate the possibility that the person might be better off taking some small risks in their life. There are also some who are fearful of the elderly person's arriving on their doorstep and of having to turn them away or take them back to hospital. These are obviously legitimate and understandable concerns, and yet should the decision they lead to prevail ? This is an opinion which I, as a professional providing a service, do not want to act on, and yet if I ignore it surely I begin to weaken the whole system of consumer consultation: one might ask with some reason why I bother to ask opinions when I do not listen to them.

One answer is obviously to work hard on the ways in which we gauge the opinions of the elderly people themselves, and yet this will take some considerable effort to do in any organized way. Another answer is to increase our level of sophistication about who is a consumer of what aspect of our services. A related issue is how long after using a service a person can be defined as a 'user'. In Mental Health services, recipients are often concerned about those services and articulate about their shortcomings some time after using them, rather than at the time; and yet we need to make sure that we have up to date views on our services.

A second concern involves the choices which must be made in setting up user feedback system. Clearly this means that other issues, which may appear to be more immediately related to service quality, will receive less input, at least until such time as the investment in service user opinion pays off. The choice to invest in the feedback system therefore constitutes an act of faith in the efficacy of user involvement. Given what we know from the research about the length of time it can take to build a climate in which meaningful and coherent feedback can be elicited, (Nadler, 1977) such a decision could well be unpopular within the provider organization whose personnel are all too aware of specific service deficits which also need investment to rectify.

In a poor service I would maintain that the more obvious inadequacies of the service should be addressed before turning to the task of setting up user feedback systems. The argument for this is first, that one should tackle poor services as quickly as possible and not waste time and users energy in telling us about obvious problems about which we already know. Secondly, I would suggest that if providers are seen to be addressing at least some problems, service users are then more likely to be reassured that there is a genuine wish to improve services and that it may be worthwhile making the effort to be involved with a user feedback system. Thirdly, staff involved with the service need to face the challenge of change and develop some acceptance of it and success at it before they can make good use of users' opinions. Lastly, if the first changes demanded of an obviously poor service are initiated by consumer feedback, then managers and staff would seem to have abrogated their responsibility to monitor and improve services. In doing so they will have put consumer opinion in the awkward and unhelpful position of being the only overt source of criticism and force for change. As such, it can easily be side-lined as the organization closes ranks to resist criticism.

Using feedback

The second issue for the provider involves the use of data generated from consumer feedback. Often the feedback, by its very nature, will largely reflect direct interactions between frontline staff and the service users. Few of us genuinely welcome potentially critical feedback and there is a

100

very real danger that users views will adversely affect staff morale, especially if the people concerned feel that they alone are being criticized. This is even more likely if staff feel that the faults in their service are caused by factors outside their control and that there are a great many faults. The provider management, therefore, needs to ensure first that feedback is known to involve all levels of the organization; secondly, that the staff organization is such that potentially critical feedback can be received without undue feelings of being attacked; and thirdly, that the feedback is in a form which can lead to useful action. While there is a need for feedback to be freely expressed by the service users so that their views can be heard fully, those views must be 'processed' or at least monitored to ensure that the information reaches the right staff in a useful format that can then lead to useful service changes. This will involve not only attention to the form and content of feedback given and to its target group, but also some careful thought about the mechanisms through which staff can then change their service delivery. In other words, the implementation of user feedback systems needs careful management if it is to give staff the context in which they might respond to the information given. These arrangements have to be made in some detail so that users can comment freely and staff in their turn can be free to respond with innovation. The creation of this environment is the responsibility of the service managers and it can be just as difficult to achieve as the initial securing of accurate feedback.

One illustration of this is the case of a ward where I once worked. The service provided was kindly in intent but unimaginative and variable in quality. The staff group were divided in their opinions on the cause of the problems, so much so that some were unable to acknowledge that there were real problems. In this environment there was a lack of constructive debate about how to improve and all attempts to encourage such debate ran the risk of being construed as attacks. Criticisms were personalized and led to blaming among the staff. Clearly in this sort of environment, the managers need to work with the staff to develop an atmosphere in which some questioning can occur and criticism can begin to be seen as potentially constructive. This is more easily said than done. To expose this staff group to user feedback in an unstructured way would have compounded problems rather than solving them.

Service development

The two issues examined so far focus on the implementation of user feedback systems in the short and medium term. However it is quite clear that were such systems in place and working well they would also bring the potential for quite far reaching long-term implications. The indications are that users often value the way in which services are delivered rather than the specific content of the treatment package. They are likely to want to be seen promptly, feel 'understood' and to be 'treated as an individual'. Users will have views on how services should develop and indeed whether particular services develop. All this seems eminently reasonable. In recognizing how little our services currently do these things, it is easy to be overcome by our sense of guilt.

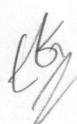

However, if we get too involved with our guilt there is a danger of missing what such changes might mean for our services. If the style of service delivery is really valued above content, for example, then users might prefer more staff with relatively less training who are able to see them promptly and take time to discuss their individual opinions, rather than to see more highly trained staff members who are, by definition, more expensive and thus available to fewer people or for more limited amounts of time. One can imagine a whole number of such scenarios which might develop from truly valuing consumer views and acting on them. This issue goes to the heart of the professional's sense of needing to take responsibility for the content of services, for judgments about how therapy should proceed and for what constitutes good practice. To what extent should these decisions be shared, and if they are given to consumers, what is the difference between a professional service and that of a helpful friend? How can we expect service users to prioritize spending on services when they are so painfully aware of specific needs for services? One partial solution to these questions might at least be to make public professional decisions about the way services are provided. This would involve 'coming clean' about issues such as our choices of what staff to employ, the content of their job descriptions, and the service targets we set.

A second potential area of difficulty raised by involving service users in service development is that they often want to develop services in ways we are not 'licensed' to do. One example of this might be the wish to increase day care services. For me as an NHS service provider this could well seem not my business since Social Services have the responsibility, and theoretically the resource for such services. Such service boundaries are rightly seen as nonsensical by many service users but they are very much part of the professionals' reality. This sort of difficulty could, of course, be met by joint finance or joint funding of services but it certainly presents service providers with an additional challenge which they may be loathe to take on. In essence, what is involved in all this is a fundamental challenge to the tradition of professionals directing services and of being acknowledged to know what is 'a good service' and what is 'best' for the consumer. At some level, staff are likely to recognize this, even if the fear of such a challenge is not clearly articulated and to resist the empowerment of users accordingly.

In summary, as a service providing professional, and latterly a general manager, the prospect of embarking on involving user opinion in our service management is both attractive and frightening. The mechanics of making such a system work well seem rather daunting. In my stronger moments I recognize that it is the long-term neglect of users' views which has led to this situation. Had we involved consumers, even a little, in years gone by, we would now be in a much better position to get meaningful feedback and implement decisions based on it. The stress placed on involving service users by our government has kicked us into doing so but it also places great stress on doing so fast and well. In this situation, opinion tends to polarize and professionals who were once all-powerful feel powerless. In fact, of course, neither extreme is to be encouraged. As service providers, we need to develop a variety of ways of eliciting users' views so as to give a balanced and richer assessment of the service, and a variety of ways of reviewing and developing our services on the small and the larger scale. These developments need to be guided by service managers so that the structures are in place which allow the content of services to be influenced by those they serve.

12 Contracting for mental health services: The place of users' views

James Raftery

This paper explores how District Health Authorities might include patients' views in their purchasing strategies, drawing on two sources of experience. First, the work currently being undertaken at the Department of Health (as part of Project 26) to provide assistance to commissioning authorities on a nationwide basis. The second relates to the experience of a single health district, Wandsworth Health Authority, which has been working in this area for over several years.

The tone of much of the discussion of consumer feedback continues as it was prior to the NHS reforms. Many people have not come to terms with the radical changes which provide new powerful levers for change in every health authority – namely the contracting process. In purchasing scope exists for gathering patients' views and including them in contract specification, for specifying future monitoring, and for targeting improvements. There are also limitations, particularly in the availability of tools. We need methods which can be taken off-the-shelf and applied to the mental health sector.

The NHS reforms which separate purchasing and providing functions fit well with the increasing expectation that consumer views be included in the planning and management of health care. The Patients' Charter (HMSO, 1991) has set basic standards to be met by the NHS, for example, in relation to waiting times. A demand for high basic standards of consumer service plus greater involvement, characterizes attitudes as we move towards the end of the century. A revolution has occurred in service industries concerning the importance of quality, the role of technology, and of competition, quality of personal service in health services, is increasingly linked to health outcome.

A number of features related to the role of the consumer apply particularly to the British health care system:

- the NHS ranks low by international standards on consumer satisfaction (Leitman *et al*, 1991);
- the NHS is a product of war-time and post-war queuing;
- capitation funding is less consumer orientated than fee for service systems.

The contracting process

Figure 1 summarizes the process of contracting, linking the contract, service specification in the contract and a purchasing plan for the district. The current baseline of services provides the starting point against which progress can be measured.

This process can result in a specification of the service largely as it was prior to the contracting service, with minor tuning of services; or in some service modifications; or in fundamental reviews. The challenge is to include the role of the consumer in this overall process. Efforts to include consumer and patient views might be strategically located by focusing on services with high levels of use, cost or general concern. Unfortunately, very few examples exist now that this is being carried out in practice.

One reason for this may be the complexities and difficulties inherent in the overall process of contracting for health services generally. Work for the Department of Health on the purchasing role of health authorities has suggested three key elements to their purchasing plans:

- epidemiological needs assessment;
- a comparative perspective;
- a corporate view.

Currently, both services and information about them are packaged in unhelpful ways, for example, by specialities or client groups. In order to have a more precise view of needs and services purchasers require information and classifications on a disease-specific basis. The 'burden of disease' approach can inform a rational approach to the assessment of needs and the allocation of resources to competing claims for service.

There are contrasting facets to the burden of mental illness imposed on the community. Mental illness accounts for very few life years lost, although there could be some misclassification in the figures. In terms of morbidity as measured by days off work, mental illness appears to impose a high burden. The most striking feature of the costs is that mental illness is the single most expensive disease by a long way, accounting for 22% of total NHS expenditure (including mental handicap, with accounts for about one third of that, leaving 15% of all NHS spending being on mental health services). One reason for this is the cost of long-term inpatients. Unpacking this overall mental health expenditure one might use Goldberg & Huxley's (1980) model of filtering the proportions of persons referred for psychological disorders. The services used at different levels within primary and secondary care can be established along with estimates of their costs. This type of service costing process has not really been attempted hitherto but such mapping of patterns of service use and costs offers districts a way of clarifying both what they currently purchase as well as what changes might be appropriate.

The next step is to translate these patterns of service use and costs into service specifications. At this point it becomes possible to insert not only what we know about cost effectiveness but also where the maximum benefits might be and to include user views within that. In a review undertaken at the York Centre for Health Economics, O'Donnell (1988) identified only seven studies of cost effectiveness carried out in the UK psychiatric services. Most of these have been with outpatients, CPN, alternatives to inpatient hospitalization and different models of services. This suggests that we should employ great caution in how far we feel able to base improved service specification on this form of empirical study.

Including users' views

One can begin to ask who (how?) best to employ consumer feedback as a tool for specifying services. A number of issues arise. Firstly, the numbers of patients involved varies. For example, with in-patients these are relatively small, about 1,000 in a year (for one average district), whereas for GP consultations it may be as high as 57,500. There may also be some trade-offs involved: does one wish to specify satisfaction with the service or to increase the level of case finding and diagnostic pick-up at the primary care level? Purchases must make complex judgements between level of spending, what is known about cost-effectiveness of that spending, the numbers of patients who are going through the service, what controls exist and where it may be most appropriate to take patient views into account.

Perhaps too, to varing degrees one might want to include patients' views depending on the nature of the disease and its severity. For example, in an Accident and Emergency department it may be more important to consider technical and response time considerations than patient satisfaction. However, in the case of a chronic condition with regular repeated consultations, patient satisfaction may be more important, relating to the surroundings, the way one is treated as a person and

Issues.

107

so on. This may also relate to such issues as the duration and the intensity of the contact that the patient has with the services.

Contracting offers a means of ensuring that user views are systematically recorded and utilized in redesigning services. The experience with one typical district service illustrates of a beginning to this process, although since msot of the work did not focus on mental health services much more remains to be done in respect of these services.

Wandsworth Health Authority

The starting point for this work was that, as a part of its 'corporate view' of the services which it wished to see provided, Wandsworth Health Authority had developed the following quality goals:

- to provide health care in a manner acceptable to each patient and client;

- to treat each patient and client with dignity and respect;

- to encourage staff to maintain the highest quality of care;

- to inform each patient of what treatment can be provided and to share the decision on the choice of treatment.

Adopted by the Health Authority in 1988, these goals are displayed prominently on walls in public areas and are reflected in the health authority's mission statement. The aim is to empower both those who wish to complain and those staff who want to bring about change. A firm and public commitment by the relevant purchasing authority should be a foundation for bringing in the user perspective to services. This general commitment will in future be built in to the contract for services for all providing agencies.

Establishing the views of users in Wandsworth took a variety of forms, including:

- a qualitative/investigative study, using interviews and groups;

- household survey (1,200 people);

- patient satisfaction survey;

- GP survey;

- survey of long-stay psychiatric inpatients.

The first of these studies was a preliminary one undertaken using qualitative methods by a commercial organization, the Specialist Research Unit (SRU), which undertook a large number (about 200) of group discussions with users of the health service and spent considerable time interviewing decision makers in the hospital. A commercial organization, used to doing work in the private sector, SRU were startled by their findings on the NHS. One major difference had to do with the academic atmosphere which characterized thinking in the teaching hospital, where problems tended to be discussed and analysed rather than acted upon.

Main findings of the qualitative study included:

- people were satisfied with medical care but were not with personal care;

- official complaints are only the tip of the iceberg;

- there was an age cohort effect, with younger people less satisfied;

- providers were also dissatisfied about some aspects of the service.

Subsequently, Wandsworth HA carried out a household survey of 1,200 people in an attempt to put more precise scales to the dimensions that had come out of this qualitative work. It also hoped to track people's patterns of service usage both in relation to patients preferences and proximity of service.

Results varied by electoral ward and in relation to which hospital of the four people had used (and some patients felt they were not given a choice). In the survey 37% had been outpatients in the last year. Of these, half had late appointments at outpatients and 20% (of 37%) had to wait more that two hours.

Other results were related to specific aspects of the service. With respect to general practice: 15% would have liked to change GP; many would be happy to have the practice nurse carry out basic tasks. General health questions followed up an earlier study: 35% claimed to be fit and healthy but smoked; lower socio-economic groups felt less capable of preventing illness.

Day surgery and travel questions showed that: 16% had a day operation; but around half favoured an overnight stay; 80% of people supported day surgery if there was good backup from District Nurses; people were prepared to travel to cut waiting time (especially young/affluent groups) but were not keen to cross the Thames. Turning to who was caring for others the survey found: 4% were currently caring mainly for elderly people on low incomes. Most of these wanted more home care. In relation to publications: 60% were unaware of Wandsworth Health Authority News (which was distributed free to all households) but client specific publications were better known.

Perhaps not surprisingly, people were keen to use locally-accessible services such as the teaching hospital in an adjacent district, even when these did not conform to delineated mental health catchment areas. Thus user preferences can raise tricky issues about contracting for mental health services in relation to the current consensus in favour of organization of mental health services on a catchment-area basis.

In relation to issues of patient satisfaction with acute hospital services, Wandsworth chose to take a readily-available model – the CASPE approach (Heckels, Chapter 4) which we took the opportunity to evaluate and to modify. It was hoped to attain a higher response rate (50% in CASPE) and by using personal interviewers a 68% response rate was achieved. In addition, the survey followed up a cohort of ex-inpatients (23%) for narrative accounts. Some extra questions were also added. The results showed wide variations by question and by hospital ward.

The highest levels of satisfaction were with medical and nursing care. The lowest levels were for domestic services, information and parking. Follow-up interviews showed that the inpatient questionnaire worked well and suggested that future questionnaires should pay greater attention to the interpersonal aspects of care. It is also important to note that more dissatisfaction emerged in personal accounts than in the questionnaire responses.

The survey results have been used us a baseline in contracting. The DHA as a purchaser is now much more concerned with Wandsworth residents and is using its contracting power to bring about changes. In particular the DHA is specifying improvements in contracts concerning cleanliness, provision of information, and complaint procedures, all of which arose from the surveys. Finally, the DHA is now planning to use the same patient satisfaction survey in the 4 main provider hospitals to assess needs and changes.

We used the Critical Incident Technique (Jones, Chapter 3) and followed up one third of the patients who had completed the patient satisfaction survey. The results of this work (Raftery and Zarb, 1990) demonstrated that, in terms of method, it was important to have interviewers ensuring that people did fill in the questionnaire and that helping them to do so boosted the response rate from 50 to about 70%. We did not demonstrate any difference between responders and non-responders. Perhaps not surprisingly, in the follow-up interview work, it was apparent that people were enormously relieved to have someone to talk to even though they were reasonably satisfied with the service. It was found that patients were capable of making acute distinctions, for example, between agency and non-agency nurses. We concluded that, although it is right to approach the issue with a simple survey technique, there is a lot of scope for further development and fine tuning. Additionally, it is important to follow up the work to ensure that one is measuring the right things.

The final piece of work undertaken was a survey carried out in the mental health unit in Wandsworth by MacDonald *et al* (1988) who were commissioned to get the views of the long-stay psychiatric inpatients. This survey showed that while patients were generally satisfied, significant variations existed by hospital ward. Factors causing greatest dissatisfaction included failure to be treated as individuals and feelings of isolation and apathy. There was a 73% response rate and a principal components analysis identified a number of significant factors accounting for dissatisfaction. Although this is one of the most difficult groups to obtain views from, this work demonstrated that it was not only possible to get their views but that the views identified meaningful and important issues in the service and with management commitment, they could be addressed.

Conclusion

All of these pieces of work were undertaken in the context of the old structures. I see much more opportunity now to bring about change through contracting than previously. Formerly, one might do the survey but be left complaining the managers took no notice. Having made the separation between purchaser and provider, it becomes clear that the only way to bring about change on the provider side is by not being aggressive. The purchasers need to be clear about what they want, to begin to identify a strategy of change involving specific individuals and to try to win some of the 'high ground' in the argument.

As a purchaser, one is being made responsible for money in order to improve the health of the population and to make the service more responsive. It is important, therefore, to capture the high ground rather than leaving it to the clinicians or to the pressure groups. If they can be brought in subsequently, so much the better. There has never been more opportunity to work for change in this way.

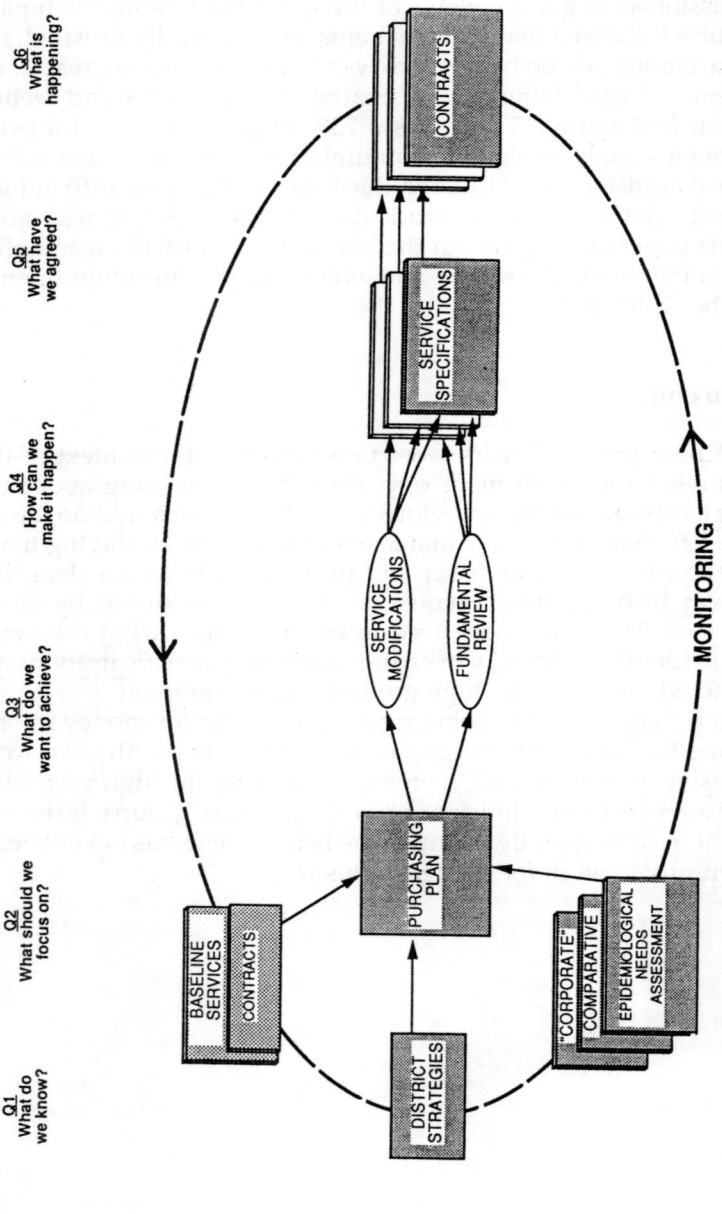

Figure 1 The Contracting Process

13 Purchasing for people

Ingrid Barker

Newcastle District Health Authority is taking a consumer-led approach to its purchasing activity. Here it is argued that user participation is vital to the success of the purchasing role and the achievement of relevant contracts for services. Newcastle's own progress in establishing consumer groups to inform purchasers and some indications given of future directions will be described in this chapter.

Centrality of consumerism to the NHS & Community Care Act

'Our experiences have led us to pose the question: If these services are for our own good why do we feel so bad about them?' (Beeforth, 1990). The service users who wrote in these terms might have been encouraged by the then Prime Minister's claim in the foreword of *Working for Patients*, 'We aim to extend patient choice... All the proposals in this White Paper put the needs of the patients first' (HMSO, 1989). Indeed, the very title of the White Paper declares the centrality of the service user to the reforms. The platforms on which users have campaigned – access, choice, information, redress and representation (Potter, 1988) – are evident in both *Caring for People* and *Working for Patients*. The concern to redress the imbalance of power between those who provide and those who use services must be reflected in purchasing as a key activity within an NHS charged with responding to the needs of users. Indeed, the role of the purchaser requires a Copernican revolution in our thinking – no longer are the needs and demands of services themselves the centre of the District Health Authority universe but the needs and demands of people who use those services.

The government's own publications often speak of 'consumerism', yet the term 'consumerism' is itself misleading. Too often the NHS is guilty of confusing customer relations or PR which keeps people as passive recipients of a service, with consumerism which is more radical in nature. In his classic consumerist text, *Unsafe at Any Speed*, Nader (1965) describes consumerism as the collective activity of concerned citizens in exposing negative aspects of organizations. Together citizens gather information, publicise it, litigate and thereby seek change. They may have paid organizers and may use the help of 'ethical whistle blowers' within the organization in order to bring to account an unaccountable executive. Nader shows how this approach forced change in a major car company which would otherwise have continued to manufacture dangerous cars. This style of consumerist activity, which is perhaps most akin to community action, is probably not what most purchasers have in mind. Some may assume that it is not even possible to engage people in this way. A consumer may be defined as an informed individual who has choice and purchasing power. Many of the most disadvantaged people who are likely to have disproportionately high need for mental health services lack information, choice or the resources to buy even the basics in life. The challenge of democracy itself, however, is to search for mechanisms by which disadvantaged people can express and exercise their views in a way which is constructive for the dominant values in our society.

The centrality of purchasing/contracting to the Act

If consumerism is central to the NHS Act then so is purchasing. Despite the flurry of interest around the establishment of Trusts and GP fundholders, the really big change to the system is the purchaser/provider split and the contractual relationship which flows from that. District Health Authorities are becoming increasingly free from management responsibilities for provider units and are required to:

- assess the needs of the population for health care;

- prioritize use of money in relation to need;

- decide what services will most appropriately meet those needs;

- place contracts with providers for the right sort of services;

- monitor the quality and effectiveness of the services.

So in what way can consumerism in Nader's sense be seen as central to purchasing? DHAs charged with the responsibility to purchase services on behalf of the local population are failing in their duty if they are not promoting collective activity by people who use the services. Given the non-elected status of the new DHA members, it is unsatisfactory to argue that the Authority itself makes the purchasing organization accountable. The purchaser's credibility and authority must be derived from its effectiveness in involving consumers in every aspect of its activity. Indeed, the Management Executive exhorts, 'True consumer involvement is more than just a consultation exercise to 'rubber stamp' a decision the DHA has, in effect, already taken' (NHSME, 1991). Shifting power in favour of service users means enabling their participation in real decision making.

Acting on this will bring benefits to purchasers and users alike. Consumer support will brighten the chances of DHAs winning the public argument about prioritizing of resources in the face of anxious and vocal consultants. Service users can bring a unique knowledge and expertise to purchasing. They can provide information about the nature of need and the extent of needs that are not met, they can understand which quality measures will really make a difference to patients, they can be in the best position to monitor some aspects of the services and they can bring a fresh perspective to planning for future services.

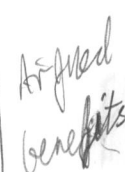

Factor working against user involvement in purchasing

It is often said that 'every problem is an opportunity'. For some, user involvement in purchasing is an 'insurmountable opportunity'. There are real factors working against it.

a) DHAs are already relating to large populations and some are merging to create mega purchasing organizations. These DHAs will find it difficult to avoid 'planning services for populations they are not in contact with and that they do not know'.

b) Particularly where there is a monopoly provider, there will be pressure on purchasers from the provider/professional view of what is 'best' for people. Recently a DGM said to a Trust Manager, 'Next year we may want to buy crumpets not bread'. The Trust Manager replied. 'Then we will have to tell you that crumpets are poisonous and bad for people'.

c) The culture of DHAs is dominated by acute sector considerations. The community care groups' interest in user involvement is therefore not often reflected in DHA thinking.

d) DHAs face financial constraints which make it difficult for them to find money to spend on user groups or to put extra cash into the sorts of services users would value.

e) Many user groups have yet to understand the opportunity which purchasing offers to bring about change.

Yet at a meeting of the national network of mental health purchasers, most of the forty or so purchasers represented were keen to make user involvement happen!

The Newcastle Mental Health Consumer Group

Newcastle DHA has been pressing forward with a consumerist approach to purchasing and has made some early progress in the field of mental health. A consumer group has been formed at the initiative of provider and purchaser who share the costs and benefits of the group. Consisting of 15 service users and carers, this small group is developing a much wider network of contacts and the broad constituency of users will elect members after the first year so that the group becomes more democratic. It has a paid facilitator and a grant which enables a small honorarium to be paid to each member. The honorarium recognises the principle of valuing the members' work and the extent of time they devote. The consumer group is therefore not a free good but at £37,000 per year is a significant cost both to the DHA and the provider. Before committing such sums to similar groups in other fields the mental health group will be carefully evaluated by the DHA.

The role of the consumer group in relation to purchasing is fourfold:

- contributing to needs assessment, particularly using anecdotal evidence;

- suggesting quality measures which will make a real difference to users to be incorporated into contracts;

- monitoring the performance of contracts particularly in relation to quality;

- contributing to planning for future services.

The early signs are promising. Members have been involved in revising the draft specifications for contracts, identifying and prioritizing appropriate quality measures and will have a monitoring role in relation to some of these measures. The mental health contracts therefore have some clients-eye views on the service. For example, one quality measure specifies that all patients must have their own toothbrushes and their own underwear and outer clothing. Without user views, purchasers would have assumed that such basic requirements were already met.

As part of its monitoring role the group is undertaking a series of visits to both the ESMI/EMI services and the Rehabilitation and Continuing Care services purchased for Newcastle. Members had just reported to purchaser on their findings and will submit a full report after six months.

116

All eight contract areas will eventually be covered thus offering the purchaser information about the service form the viewpoint of those it is aimed to help.

The consumer group is also to be involved in developing an understanding of need and consequently, of what kind of service should be purchased to meet that need. A group of purchasing stakeholders has been convened. Consisting of representatives of the DHA, Social Services, CHC, GPs and with a majority drawn from the consumer group, this 'Purchasing for People' meeting is reviewing the mental health strategy for the city in partnership with providers. Already it is challenging the existing plans for acute mental health services. Familiar user demands for 24 hour crisis services and safe houses are being brought to the table and are being met with accord from the GPs and other stakeholders. This will have a huge influence on the purchasing intentions for future years. Thus services users are involved in the powerful activities of purchasing - needs assessment and service planning.

Since user involvement is already in vogue in mental health it is arguable that Newcastle has begun with the easiest client group. Yet if a group of people widely regarded as unreliable and of doubtful credibility and who have experienced profound loss of personal power can take an opportunity to influence purchasing then it must be possible for others to do so.

In this belief, Newcastle DHA is establishing consumer groups in the fields of physical disability, elderly, learning difficulties and HIV/AIDS. All these groups will have a role in needs assessment, establishing and monitoring quality measures and in developing ideas for future services. Again, it could be argued that these priority care groups are reasonably well organized and represent the simpler tasks. The big challenge will be to take these consumerist activities into the acute sector.

In some areas this should not be a herculean task. Specialties such as obstetrics with associated user organizations such as Maternity Alliance or National Childbirth Trust, or ophthalmology with its range of voluntary organizations relating to sight, are ripe for picking. Many chronic conditions such as back pain or diabetes also have well established self-help groups who could be engaged in purchasing. Here the challenge is for a shift in our thinking to enable known user groups to be given an opportunity for involvement.

Large, diffuse specialties with a quick throughput such as general surgery will be more difficult to tackle, but even here, in the lair of customer relations tools such as surveys and questionnaires, it is possible to involve service users more actively. Short-term 'focus groups' where groups of patients speak about their experiences of the service will identify which are the really important issues to tackle in a questionnaire. It should also be possible to set up public meetings around some of the specific topics raised since large numbers of people will have had some contact with the service.

All this is a long way from the cynicism with which the reforms are viewed by some. I have heard them say that the new NHS with its undemocratic structures, its philosophy of cost-cutting over quality, presents a threat to consumer participation and choice. It is vital that purchasing DHAs counter this with a consumerist approach to ensure that the reforms do indeed work for patients.

14 The role of pressure groups in creating change

Liz Sayce

Independent of both purchaser and provider organizations is a range of independent or quasi-independent groups which aim to produce change in public services. These bodies are not necessarily user groups and may have a mixture of users and professionals, operating at local or national level but with a legitimate claim to have a separate voice. Probably the most visible are national pressure groups. When Douglas Hurd was Home Secretary he said that pressure groups were strangling the policy process in a serpent-like fashion (Baggott, 1988), thus preventing MPs and ministers from making decisions in the public interest. This implies a measure of influence, although there is some evidence that, in fact, the power of pressure groups over the last ten years has been declining and Baggott (1988) discusses four reasons for this. Firstly, a large parliamentary majority means that the government has no real need to listen to pressure groups at a national level. Secondly, the government has reduced its dependency on the consent or support of pressure groups by, for instance, employing its own advisors or setting up its own think tank and bypassing the consultation process. Thirdly, direct disagreement between government policy and the ideas of some pressure groups means, for example, that an organization like the Child Poverty Action Group, which consistently argues that the poorest tenth of the population is getting poorer, is going to come into head-on conflict with the government (although that is not to say that the CPAG has lost its influence). Fourthly, there has been an increasing emphasis on conviction rather than consultative politics. In this context pressure groups have lost some credibility but this does not mean they have no potential or no impact. Since the 1992 general election the Government's parliamentary majority has been reduced from 87 to 21. Also, although some pressure groups have declined, the decline has been selective; others have grown and Friends of the Earth, for example, now has 65 times more members than it had 20 years ago. Clearly, in some areas pressure groups have increased their influence.

In mental health, the issue of political conflict is not so clear cut because there is a convergence between left and right regarding community care and on some issues like devolving power to the individual. Whilst the different sides mean different things by these concepts, there are points of convergence and cross cuts between policies. In terms of mental health pressure groups at national level, there has not been an obvious decline in activity but there have been changes in the configurations of where influence is held. This chapter will put a slightly optimistic gloss on developments which may be open to different interpretations.

In the mid 1980s there was a strong lobby for stopping the hospital closure programme which, to some extent, was based on an improbable alliance between the profession of psychiatry which was trying to protect its power base; the trade unions who were concerned about their members' jobs (and were part of the labour movement which saw not closing hospitals as a way to protect the NHS); relatives' groups whose hard-pressed members were afraid of having extra responsibilities placed upon them if the hospitals were run down; and a campaigning journalist who created SANE (Schizophrenia a National Emergency) and created a rallying call around the pressure to stop the hospital closure programme. At that time MIND, which was in favour of hospital closure, and the National Schizophrenia Fellowship were openly at loggerheads in the trade press. As a result of some of that pressure, government policy shifted slightly off the course of hospital closure and in 1988 Health Circular HC(88)43 stated that hospitals should not close unless comprehensive community services were in place; and the more recent care programme approach circular HC(90)23 says that if, when somebody is assessed and when discharge is being considered, there are not resources in the community the individual should be offered the continuation of a hospital place. This could in effect mean perpetuating the existence of hospital places in the absence of community resources.

It seems then that the lobby had some success. However, opposing currents have developed more recently. In the early 1990s the user movement has grown enormously in strength and also in terms of national coordination with Survivors Speak Out and the UK Advocacy Network. Some key unions have become much more in favour of hospital closure and certainly COHSE has written very positively about community care. The new merged COHSE, NUPE and NALGO might well be quite a strong force on this issue in the future. In terms of MIND and the National Schizophrenia Fellowship, MIND has been giving more attention to carers and the National Schizophrenia Fellowship to users; MIND and NSF have collaborated on some national and local projects; and they are no longer at loggerheads, although obviously there are still differences of policy. There have been some results of this changed configuration. For example Stephen Dorrell spoke in 1991 (DoH press

120

release) of the grotesquely inappropriate allocation of resources, with well over half of the mental health budgets going into hospital care, a situation that he wanted to see significantly changed. The 1991 Green Paper, *Health of the Nation*, (HMSO, 1991) had as one of its targets for mental health the closure of many of the psychiatric hospitals by the year 2000. The closure of all the psychiatric hospitals by the year 2000 was a call made by MIND's National Director at the 1990 MIND annual conference, which suggests some direct pressure group influence at work from the pro-planned hospital closure side. Although the 1992 White Paper, the *Health of the Nation*, removed the specific target date for hospital closure, it did maintain a strong focus on replacing institutional care by comprehensive local mental health services (HMSO, 1992); and a national mental health task force, headed by David King, was established, charged with the remit of pushing that policy through on the ground.

Baggott (1988) points out that pressure groups can succeed if they have strong organization and strategy, if they are prepared to form lobbies with other groups and if they have public support. Public support is clearly a thorny issue in mental health. A study by Shula Ramon found some shift, between 1985 and 1990, in media presentations of mental health: scaremongering pieces about community care became slightly less common, and conversely positive coverage of the potential of people with mental health problems to live outside hospital was more in evidence (Ramon, 1991). It does appear from reading the press cuttings that are taken daily at MIND that there has been some more attention to people's rights, to positive representations of community living over the last two years than there was in the mid 1980s although obviously there is a long way to go. Some journalists seem concerned to take up the views of people who use services rather than adopting a scaremongering approach; and to convey the message that mental distress can affect anyone. This type of positive development helps to break down unhelpful barriers and overcome people's fear.

I shall look at the basis on which an organization like MIND, or any other pressure group which is not a user group, has any mandate to be pressurizing about anything. Before that I will describe some of the things that MIND has, even in these relatively inauspicious times, achieved nationally. In 1991, MIND succeeded in securing an amendment to the Criminal Justice Bill which means that courts have to consider the likely effect of imprisonment on somebody who appears to have a mental disorder, so that it should no longer be the case that people who are very distressed go into prisons without anybody assessing the impact of that imprisonment. There are many other things that are needed for diversion out of custody to work effectively but this is a helpful step forward.

The parliamentary social services committee in 1990 took on many service away from a primarily medical concept and towards more co-ordination of social policies and more user involvement. They also included specific recommendations in line with MIND's evidence like more bridging finance. The government gave a rather inadequate response but the health committee (as it became) used further MIND evidence to respond, thereby shifting the terms of official debate.

MIND lobbied the Department of Health on the Guidance relating to the NHS and Community Care Act 1990. Many of the things that MIND wanted to change, like having a completely independent inspectorate, the department has not changed. Some things did change, for example, the original drafts had no options for user involvement in the inspection process at all whereas now user groups are mentioned as participants in advisory committees. It is not mandatory but mention in the guidance is some progress. Another example is on the care programme approach, where MIND argued that it should not be the consultant psychiatrist who decided when somebody still needed hospital care or whether it was realistic for them to be 'treated in the community'. Now the consultant psychiatrist does not need to make that decision, so at local level people could be pushing for others to be making it: the user her/himself with input from the people who know the user's situation best, such as community based housing workers, social workers, and relatives and friends.

At local level, MIND has been identifying the demands in the Mental Health Act Code of Practice for written procedures in local authorities and health authorities. There are a number of procedures that have to be in place under the Code of Practice which some health and local authorities appear not to be aware of: for example, for local authorities there should be procedures on after care (with health authorities and voluntary organizations), availability and use of interpreters; for health authorities on providing information to patients, use of restraint and behaviour modification programmes. We surveyed authorities in the North West and found that almost no local authorities had policies on availability and use of professional interpreters and almost none had procedures on behaviour modification programmes (Shepherd, 1990). MIND uses surveys as a way of embarrassing people, highlighting the fact that things are not happening, and acting as an impetus for change. We have done similar work on the levels of registration for voting amongst users in psychiatric hospital. For example, in the North West levels rose between 1987 and 1990 from 4% to 8% (Dyer, 1990).

As well as exerting pressure directly, MIND assists others to do so. For example, we are painfully aware of the lack of information users receive about proposed treatments: the MIND/Roehampton survey of 500 users of services found 80% were dissatisfied with the information provided by the psychiatrist (MIND, 1990). For some, the first they know of treatment risks – such as tardive dyskinesia – is when they begin to develop the symptoms. We respond by providing independent information in the form of leaflets, fact-sheets and rights guides, based on which, some users tell us they have been able successfully to argue to see their records or to have their medication reduced.

We also provide policy materials which people can use to push for change locally: for example, MIND's Policy on Case Registers was recently passed by a local MIND group to an NHS mental health service manager, with the result that the local policy changed to allow informed consent to having one's name on the register; and MIND's policy on User Involvement was welcomed by the NHS Management Executive and disseminated via regional health authorities to local units.

MIND also provides legal advice and representation, and support in making complaints. MIND was involved in unearthing some of the truth about the death of Bridget Brosnan in the Lister Hospital, Stevenage: a verdict of unlawful killing was returned following evidence of excessive levels of medication and bruising on her body. Sometimes supporting users or staff in making a complaint can change practice: a nurse who contacted MIND decided he did not want to make public the excessive level of constraint he had witnessed (5 hours for an elderly woman, tied into a 'geriatric chair'); but with MIND's support he did complain through the line management system and the practice stopped in two days.

Finally, sometimes MIND pulls together and focuses activities at national, local and individual level to maximize pressure for change. In July 1992 MIND launched a one-year campaign to improve mental health services for women (MIND, 1992). Called 'Stress on Women', its aims included increased choice and safety for women users: for instance, to ensure women can opt for women-only space in hospitals and other facilities, to promote policies to prevent and tackle sexual harassment and abuse in the services, and to raise awareness of differential treatments given to women and to men (and indeed to different groups of women, depending on factors such as race, age and social class). Four months into the campaign it had the backing of organizations including the Equal Opportunities Commission, the Royal College of General Practitioners, the Transcultural Psychiatry Society and the Royal College of Nursing. Both Tim Yeo, MP and Duncan Nichol, Chief Executive of the NHS Management Executive, had commented favourably on the campaign; and the Royal College of Psychiatrists had agreed to re-examine its policy supporting mixed wards. Questions had been raised in Parliament; and radio, TV and press had covered the campaign, with the result that many women spoke out for the first time on the taboo subject of abuse and harassment within psychiatric settings. MIND also produced a leaflet on 'your right to say no'. A member of MINDLINK, MIND's user a leaflet on 'your right to say no'. A member of MINDLINK, MIND's user network, spoke about the campaign to women patients in Ashworth Hospital (a regime that had just been condemned by the Inquiry as 'infantilizing, demeaning and anti-therapeutic for women') (HMSO, 1992) and eight women from Ashworth subsequently attended a seminar outside the hospital, where one commented that 'it was nice to be treated as an equal'.

Through all these means, MIND uses its influence to push for greater power and choice for users.

What then is the basis on which an organization like MIND does this pressuring kind of work, given that pressure groups could be formed from people from any power base? The Royal College of Psychiatrists is a pressure group and it is currently using that position to argue that mental health resources should be spent on an increase in the number of consultant psychiatrists. It is legitimate to ask whether they have asked users if they think that is the best use of the available resources. For an organization like MIND, and other organizations that are not user oriented such as community health councils or 'watch dogs', the Mental Health Act Commission, or Health Advisory Service, it seems to me that they are worth their salt if they are pushing for user involvement in those services with which they are in contact. A health service inspection should be inspecting for the existence of effective user involvement in the services – that should be very high on the agenda of activities. Such organizations of course, need to be accountable to users and need to ensure that as an organization they are actually taking up the issues concerning users. MIND has agreed a policy on user involvement which applies both to MIND and to other mental health services and we have set up an audit process to look at the quality of MIND's local association services, including the levels of user involvement. MIND still has much progress to make in involving users and it is an issue we grapple with constantly. We do involve users formally in decision making, and in addition we increasingly have users on the staff and on council of management, who are not there as user representatives but who bring a user perspective. We have also done qualitative and quantitative research into users' views, like the *People First Survey* (MIND, 1990). MIND also takes up the issues people bring to us through our information lines and our legal department. Some of the functions that MIND currently undertakes and the activities of organizations like CHCs will increasingly be done by user organizations and I would like to see that balance shifting, but broad-based pressure groups are not redundant at this point in history.

15 Training mental health providers in the 1990s

Dr Shulamit Ramon

Considerable changes are taking place in the British mental health system both at an organizational level, with the introduction of the purchaser/provider split and at the service level with the contraction of hospital provision and the development of an alternative service system. Of particular importance for training has been the increased visibility of users' and relatives' organizations and their emerging power to exert pressure, as well as their potential to work in partnership, which have already led to a growing emphasis on establishing enabling and empowering services. At the same time the relative increase in the number of unqualified workers and the decrease in the number of qualified staff means that there is an unparalleled opportunity to develop the kind of training initiatives which are based on user empowerment and enable staff to deliver the services users want in a valuing and empowering manner.

Underpinning these changes is the belief that people in mental distress, however severe, would be best served in the community and by being supported to have an ordinary life as far as is possible. In many ways, the current changes are as radical as were the changes which took place in the aftermath of the Second World War, even though underlying contradictory motivations can be detected now – as then (Scull, 1978; Ramon, 1985; Biggs, 1990; Holloway, 1991). To ensure that this radical change is indeed implemented, the content and the format of training on offer to qualified and unqualified workers within the mental health system should reflect the best in the attitudes, knowledge and skills which follow from this shift. This paper will focus primarily on qualified professionals, and will address training needs related to working with the continuing care client.

The content of training

The focus on providing services in the community in the least institutionalizing settings and the most conducive to fostering an ordinary life has a number of implications for professional good practice.

In relation to attitudes, the client's and the carer's versions of a situation are as valid as that of the professional. Consequently, both should be active partners in decisions concerning intervention. For such an approach to prevail, the view of the client as ill and unable to exercise proper judgement has to change to a view which recognizes that clients are able, for most of the time, to participate in decision making and to take responsibility for their own lives, even though they may require continuous support. Services should be provided in non-segregating settings, and as much as possible within universal, non-stigmatising services, and offer opportunities for social valorization of the service users. Given the objectives which lie behind the changes, psychosocial factors and psychosocial methods of intervention are of at least equal importance to medical perspectives.

In relation to knowledge, an understanding of clients' and carers' views on what is mental distress for them, and which are the best means to prevent and alleviate it, is essential for professionals. Knowledge of decision-making processes is necessary at a variety of levels, such as the individual, the family, the sub-culture and the organization in which the professional is working. Knowledge of the impact of institutionalization, its prevention, and the creation of opportunities for social valorization is required. Finally, awareness of the socio-economic, political, and psychological contexts in which people live is indispensable, and should be accompanied by knowledge of psychosocial interventions.

In terms of the skills which are necessary, it is important to be able to encourage clients and carers to express their views, individually and collectively, as well as to be able to assess the client's potential. There are important skills of fostering partnership in decision-making, of influencing organizational change and of effectively participating in such changes. It is essential to possess the skills for establishing socially valued services and for working on the impact of the damage done to users by their experience of institutionalization, condescending approaches and over-emphasis on weakness and failure. Finally, there is a range of skills required for effective psychosocial interventions, including networking.

The different professions contributing to mental health services differ in their degree of knowledge and use of psychosocial intervention methods and all are ill-equipped to encourage the expression of clients' views and to translate those into service delivery. Hence we face a major challenge as to how to introduce these areas into training, how to re-train those already practising, and how to train the trainers. The re-training aspect is particularly taxing for staff, as it involves accepting the fundamental

126

critique of a number of current professional contributions, unlearning some key approaches and practices, and re-learning a new set.

The state of current basic qualification training

Introducing relevant training here should be easy as it starts from a relatively clean slate. This may be so in the case of the trainees, but is not so in relation to the trainers or to the practice component of a course. Validating bodies of educational institutions have stressed the introduction of competence-related objectives, at the considerable neglect of conceptual and ethical issues, as well as those of policy and history. The result is that the qualifying professional knows relatively little about the context in which the changes mentioned above are taking place, understands even less about the reasons for these changes, and has not been educated to become involved in a change process. The superficial use of 'management-speak', especially around quality assurance, is only likely to lead to its repetition aimed at impressing examiners and potential employers.

At the same time, the focus on competence has increased attention to skills teaching and evaluation of actual performance, leading to greater reliance on an apprenticeship model of practice training. This model has the advantages offered by direct modelling and feedback and the disadvantage of encouraging imitation while discouraging originality and innovation. Most practice experience is gained in hospital-based services, even though the direction of the change is to limit and move away as much as possible from these services. No training concerning a general approach to change in service systems is given, even on courses which look at the policy context (such as some social work courses), and this includes a lack of training in initiating service innovation.

Likewise, with the exception of a few nursing and social work courses, no attention is paid to the collective views of users and informal carers or to how to get them involved in services. The continuing care client appears as one sub-client group on the agenda, the one about which pathology and chronicity are emphasized, and very little is presented to encourage the professional-to-be to believe that positive outcomes may be achieved with them. Often, these clients are portrayed as the people who are hard to place, difficult to work with, uncooperative, non-compliant concerning medication, and unmotivated to change. All of these stereotypes are described as part of practice wisdom, whereas positive findings from demonstration projects and rehabilitation programmes, and the methods by which they have been obtained, are rarely outlined (Mosher and Burti, 1989).

In most practice placements expectation of the clients and of working with them are low, and trainees are not encouraged to move beyond the accepted practice wisdom. In a minority of practice placements a very different attitude prevails. In teams specializing in working with this client group a much more positive approach prevails, experimentation with new ways of working takes place, and teams often take pride in their work and in their critical stance towards other services. However, these positive experiences often do not receive the reinforcement which they deserve in college. Trainees with a commitment to listening to the views and experiences of users need support and encouragement from their supervisors and tutors and will not always find that support readily available.

The state of current post qualifying training

The change in both the locus of service delivery (hospital to community) and the model (hierarchical and illness focused to multidisciplinary and empowering) is perceived by many professionals as a negative judgement on their past contribution. This is particularly noticeable within the process of hospital closure. It has been compounded by the patent lack of consultation with frontline professional providers and the introduction of new workers to manage the transitional stage, instead of acknowledging the change process as one which involves and needs all those who are part of the existing institution.

Many professionals are cynical about a system which has been starved of resources for a long time, yet went through a large number of organizational changes imposed from above. In these circumstances, attempts at service innovation tend to be perceived as yet another imposition, likely to further curtail professional autonomy. Two groups of professionals are enjoying the challenge embedded in the new directions: those who have embraced the move to managerial tasks and role definition; and those working in pioneering projects.

In-service training would ideally be the vehicle for the transmission of new approaches to service delivery and for engaging staff in the change process. However, as most in-service training opportunities tend to be very short, they are not useful tools for changing attitudes or skills, although they may add new knowledge, raise questions and doubts, and motivate some professionals to seek further training. Rarely do such courses seek to bring staff in touch with the experience that users have or to allow staff the opportunity to confront the very real pain, as well as the reward, that there might be in developing new ways of working.

The competence-based focus has, however, led to the production of some imaginative workshop-style manuals and videos (e.g. Alcock and Brown's *New Lifestyles*; or Davidson's *Take the Steam out of the Team*; *User Participation* by South-East MIND; and *the Self-Advocacy* pack produced by Survivors Speak Out). Their usefulness, however, continues to depend both on the trainer on the spot and on the presence of structures and support in the workplace which allow the process of change to be worked through. More longer post-qualifying courses are now available than before. These have come in part as a response to pressures within educational institutions to generate income and to focus on continuing education, and in part due to initiatives by main validating bodies, such as CCETSW and the ENB. Both of these organizations are in the process of establishing professional post-qualifying awards to be achieved through a mixture of practice and educational experiences, through a modular, credit-based system. More and more courses are based on practitioner-learners who study while they continue to work on a full-time basis, with time off work given for study by the employer.

The most popular courses among employers (encouraged by the government) are those focusing on management, perceived to be an area where there is a lack of well qualified staff, as none of the basic qualification training programmes prepares people to be managers. On these courses it is assumed that a business management approach is the best approach to be applied to the management of human services, an assumption which the author finds to be misleading: it does not differentiate what could be taken from a business management approach and what in fact should not be taken from it, given that the value system – and especially the use of people – differs considerably (and *should* differ) between business and human services. This wholesale adoption leads to a generation of managers quite unsuitable to manage human services in ways designed to promote partnership and empowerment. Of course, in principle there is no reason why training in mental health should not combine effective management principles within the human services with good professional practice.

The most popular courses which individual professionals opt for are those which focus on clinical methods and offer a postgraduate degree. Both the employers' and the individual professional's choices are understandable, given the focus on skills in everyday practice, and the social status attached to higher degrees. However, with some exceptions which will be mentioned below, the courses focusing on methods typically continue to focus on individuals only (or families only, or groups only) and fail to take into account the context in which professionals are working or in which clients and carers are living. Consequently, these courses lead to a further narrowing of the professional's perspective, instead of broadening it.

The exceptions include the few training programmes which are informed first and foremost by the contexts in which professionals work and clients live, as well as being interested in introducing change at both levels. Invariably, these are not only multidisciplinary in their approach,

129

but also multi-method, focus more on the clients' and carers' perspective, attempt to foster a more positive attitude towards working with the continuing care client, use the findings of demonstration projects, and encourage course participants to innovate in their work. Perhaps not surprisingly these courses are not to be found in medical or nursing schools, but in applied psychology and social work departments, or in independent settings. The involvement of users in the planning of such courses and their direct involvement as trainers helps to re-ground participants in an orientation to the users' versions of their reality so that they go back and check out the situation with users 'at home'.

Underlying obstacles to change in training orientation

We need to ask what are the obstacles which prevent basic training and most post-qualifying training from adopting a contextualized, change-orientated approach, interested in clients and carers as partners, and in providing socially valued services. Some of the difficulties lie in honouring the clinical tradition, in which disciplinary knowledge and skills are supposed to be universal and not context-bound. Furthermore, the adherents of the clinical approach in its purity tend not to see the contexts listed above as crucial for the success or failure of the clinical methods they are employing. In short, the interdependency between clinical methods and non-clinical contexts is left unrecognized.

A defensive stance against any change has also developed among professionals, including trainers, due to the sense of imposition, fear of criticism, and a wish to defend professional autonomy and power. This attitude prevents them and the trainees from examining in each case whether a proposed change should be welcomed, rejected or modified. In particular, the defensive stance is employed in relation to involving users and relatives at the levels of planning, running and evaluating services. This is the case both at the individual and the collective levels. Users' and carers' genuine participation in the service is perceived to be a threat to professional understanding and working, as it implies that hitherto the professional contribution has been either insufficient or incorrect in providing the right approach to the difficulties experienced by the client. Furthermore, given a prevailing attitude of viewing clients and carers not only as lacking in 'true' knowledge but also as predominately 'weak' people, it is difficult, if not impossible, to have to treat their views as those of partners. User involvement in particular is uncomfortable, as a number of users' groups have been critical of and angry about professional intervention.

Training programmes which incorporated users' contributions are also finding their position uncomfortable, as their continued collaboration with existing disciplines and mental health services, as well as the selective use of traditional knowledge, mean that they are 'reformist' rather than 'revolutionary' in nature, and can only partially satisfy the wishes of users' groups. Their position is doubly uncomfortable once they are identified within professional circles as promoting the kind of change in our mental health system which accommodating the users' perspective represents. Likewise, while welcoming the general direction of the changes in the mental health system, they may be critical of a number of aspects of the system and of specific directions and means of change.

Although on the surface the competence-based, skill-focused, pragmatic approach to training would seem to be open-ended and flexible, it hides the implicit ideological and conceptual frameworks on which it is based. Without making the underlying assumptions explicit, it is virtually impossible to develop a more questioning stance and to be able to be selective as to what constitutes good practice. The necessary unlearning and relearning cannot take place without a careful examination of issues which are not simply technical in nature – the 'why?' and the 'what for?' of practice. However, such a process is bound to be uncomfortable and to unearth conflicting views. It is worthwhile remembering that without a conceptual framework in which being critical is fostered, professionals will not be equipped to act as autonomous, yet interdependent, decision-makers or as innovators.

Existing opportunities for change in training orientation

Within the changing system there are a number of opportunities which can be used in leading training in the directions listed above. There is no substitute for the impact of listening to the angry messages of users and carers as a training tool but these should be channelled around specific topics and avoid voyeurism. There is no replacement for the experiential understanding of what it is like to suffer from mental distress, to be a service user or a carer. Consequently it is imperative to enable trainees to 'go through it'. Apart from listening to users and carers, working on oneself as someone in need of help and as a service user provides another useful tool. Working with clients on reconstructing their life history (through life books, through 'getting to know you' techniques, in group discussions) also offers similar benefits. Where appropriate, *solidarity* with users and carers should be encouraged as a training device, something which is especially effective at changing attitudes.

Pioneering projects should become training centres in collaboration with educational institutions. Such centres would offer both basic qualification and post-qualifying training options. This would enable the trainees to benefit from sharing in the struggles and the satisfactions of such projects. Teaching on organizational change should be accompanied by the participants carrying out their own innovation project. Such a project would provide excellent training in setting up objectives, testing feasibility, consultation with and participation by other workers, clients, carers, groups in the community, building one's own support system, planning and implementation. Such a process should follow an action research model, to enable professionals to become better at evaluating their own work and that of others (Ramon (1991); Ryan (1991); Tolkington (1991)). Given the pace of the changes, and the focus on quality control, possibilities for such projects should be in abundance. Projects would also provide an ideal tool with which to empower workers who have experienced change as imposition.

There are numerous opportunities to enhance a contextualized approach, as well as the group and community work orientation. These start by analysing the various contexts of an individual client, which will invariably illustrate that more than one context has been affected, or needs to be changed. The ecological model in social work is particularly useful as a conceptual and practice tool (Whittaker, 1986).

The growing awareness amongst professionals of the importance of the organizational context could – and should – be moved from its present negative attitude towards a more positive stance. This can happen if the change process is better understood and professionals are given tools to influence it. In turn, such a change depends on a necessary (and not inconsiderable) shift in the attitude of top management to the workforce which parallels the expectation that professional workers change their attitudes towards service users and carers. This is a move from a 'top-down' approach to one in which professionals are treated as partners in the change process.

Finally, a central role can be played by validating bodies in promoting and encouraging change in training. The Community Care Programme at CCETSW is providing a useful example in its systematic attempt to inform trainers, to encourage debate and to offer incentives to participate in fostering new directions.

It is clear that the increasing willingness to listen to and be influenced by the voice of mental health service users is part of a wider process of change which is overturning some of the basic underlying principles of past provision. The threats imposed by the rapid pace of change can force professionals to turn inward and make their approaches more rigid. The user voice can come to seem like one more attack on professional practice. Training has a vital role to play in enabling service providers to be open to the views of their clients, to work with clients for change and to value themselves more highly precisely because they value the people they are working with.

16 Promoting user feedback: District strategies for change

Dr David Somekh

In this paper I am going to compare and contrast the approach to user involvement in mental health services in two different locations, both of which I have been involved in. The first is an inner London borough with the associated problems of rate capping, disadvantage and a tradition of poor provision of community services by the statutory authorities. The project has been going now for about four years.

The other project was in a more affluent outer London borough which was coterminous with its health authority and here, the author had the opportunity to set up a quality assurance strategy, a major element of which was the promotion of user empowerment. This project has been running for about three years. While the outer London borough is more affluent and less overcrowded, in fact, for political reasons, it also has a poor record of community provision by the statutory authorities. Both locations are currently affected by the closure of the same large mental hospital situated some distance away which traditionally provided long-stay beds. As a result, there should be an improvement in local community provision as a substitute for what was previously provided at a distance. Inevitably, local political issues will affect the quality of the provision that is eventually established, but the reprovision and hospital closure programme is on target to be completed by the end of 1992.

One could describe the two projects as representing an evolutionary model in the inner London site and a strategic model at the other, but once the projects were established, it will be seen that the process of development becomes increasingly similar even if the form is somewhat different.

An evolutionary model

Approximately four years ago at the inner London site, Good Practices in Mental Health provided a development worker for a year with a brief

133

to set up a forum for mental health which would be a collaborative network between all the stakeholders in the mental health service, particularly users, voluntary agencies and representatives of the three principal statutory agencies, that is health authority, social services and local authority. The worker developed a constitution for the forum which would form the basis of an application to obtain charitable status. The hope was that within a year funding would be found for the public meetings which were quite well attended and, as a result of due consultation, the constitution was sent to the Charity Commission and charitable status granted. A co-ordination group was set up as part of the constitution to have ongoing management of the project and this group had representatives from the key groups mentioned above. The tasks for the forum were to set up user groups; to have strategy groups set up looking at all the different aspects of mental health provision whether in existence currently or not; and to define good practices and to propose a strategy for a development of good practice in that particular area, for example, women and mental health, or crisis intervention. The papers which resulted from the strategy groups would form the basis of a negotiation between the forum and the statutory agencies for a more direct input by stakeholders into the statutory planning process. Open meetings of the forum would provide the appropriate democratic basis for the election of co-ordination group members, for discussion of keynote issues and to encourage networking between stakeholders.

The primary problem was that after a year of satisfactory developments in which charitable status was obtained and the co-ordination group met regularly, the project worker had to withdraw but funding had not materialized and in fact, did not do so until more than a year later. This meant that the activity of the forum faltered as it had to be supported on a purely voluntary basis by co-ordination group members who were all busy in their own activities, whether professionals or other stakeholders. Eventually the two health authorities agreed to provide funding for the first two years and the co-ordination group, or what remnants of it survived the long wait for funding, very rapidly appointed their own development worker and one of the health authorities provided free accommodation and office facilities at minimum cost.

The development worker, who is currently beginning the third year of activity, rapidly set up user groups and was so successful in this enterprise that a self-sufficient user organization has come into being which has managed to obtain some funding for itself and is affiliated to the forum. With the help of the co-ordination group, the development worker organized a strategy on a yearly basis and a programme of education and information. Within the framework of the initial constitution, the emphasis of activities shifted somewhat and the open meetings are primarily centred round discussion of key issues in mental health, with constitutional and administrative matters relegated to the background.

Although some of the original strategy groups completed their task, the overall strategy for the forum has moved with the concurrent changes in the NHS to being an organization which primarily represents user views and supports the voluntary agencies associated with mental health. Now, after a couple of internal strategic reviews of its activity, it is set to negotiate a service contract with the appropriate health authorities in the context of the purchaser/provider split. One of the successful development projects has been the obtaining of funds for setting up advocacy co-ordinators in one of the health authorities served. A project in the pipeline is obtaining funding for a user-oriented quality assurance project which could lead to the offer of external monitoring of quality to the relevant health authorities.

In essence, the evolutionary model, once the development worker had been funded, has followed a predictable cycle of producing results. These provided further funding and a re-definition of the brief which in turn led to further results and funding and hopefully will continue to do so.

A strategic model

As far as the strategic model was concerned, three years ago, in the outer London area, a senior member of staff approached the Unit General Manager for Mental Health with the suggestion that there should be a quality assurance adviser to the Unit Management Group. After a year's research into the area, the quality adviser obtained agreement to write a strategy for mental health within the next three months, assisted by the mental health development officer and a representative each of users of the service and carers. The strategy that was developed has three main components, namely increasing staff awareness about quality, developing a flexible package of service evaluation which, with appropriate management arrangements, sets in motion a continuing quality cycle (in effect a total quality management system), and thirdly empowering consumers. The consumerism element has six criteria by which its development can be assessed and is seen as something which will need several years to be put in place fully.

These are:

- that a charter accepted both by consumers and the organization has currency;

- that consumer representation in the planning process is present on more than a tokenistic basis;

- that consumer feedback has a demonstrable effect upon service delivery;

- that advocacy is developed and available within the service;

- that an active role for the individual consumer in their care plan is accepted and implemented;
- that information about the service at every level is accessible to consumers.

In order to facilitate the development of user groups at arms' length from the statutory organization, the planning officer referred to above set up a forum committee which would represent carers, voluntary agencies and users. This forum was funded on a grant from the health authority. This actually meant that the funded forum worker was in place some months prior to the one in inner London getting appointed. The outer London forum quickly developed a cycle of regular public meetings on mental health issues attended by a large audience of workers in the statutory organizations, carers and users of the service. The forum worker also regularly attended meetings of the relevant quality strategy working group which began in September 1989 and was then named the Consumer Monitoring Group. However, the actual development of user groups was much slower than on the other site and in fact, as will be noted below, this important aspect of the project only became properly established after a further two years had elapsed.

In the meantime the quality adviser had to obtain funding for implementation of the strategy after its acceptance at the Unit Management Group and it happened that in the financial year 1990/91, that quality assurance funding was available from the Department of Health via the regional health authority. This was successfully bid for but this funding, together with a top-up from the Mental Health Unit, took some six months before it was actually available. This caused delay in the implementation of the full-time process that was supported by the quality assurance adviser, who was, effectively offering two sessions a week to co-ordinate the implementation of the strategy.

Taking stock of the implementation process so far (the beginning of 1991), it is clear that the immense changes within the NHS have interacted in a negative way with the quality change process. At the beginning of the year the QA adviser presented to the Unit General Manager a very detailed annual report of the implementation process with a bid for funding for 1991/92. However, the Commissioners of the service declined to provide additional funding, arguing that block contracts for mental health should include quality money as part of service delivery costs, that is not acknowledging that the funding requested was actually for development of the quality process rather than ongoing running costs. Similarly, QA development monies from the regional health authority were not available for a second year so that funding for 1991/92 has been provided but on a very insecure basis. It effectively means that the quality worker has only to the end of the financial year to deliver as much of the implementation process as possible. During the same time, the QA adviser (whose own responsibilities have shifted as the Unit organizes itself towards possible Trust status by 1992/93) has a half a day a week to co-ordinate the implementation activities and to attempt to ensure that there is sufficient management initiative to enable the implementation process to be successfully completed within 1992/93, probably with no additional funds. The Quality Review Team and the Unit Management Group act as prompts to management. By 1992/93 it is hoped that the clinical directorate structure, which is just coming into existence, will have established QA as a necessary part of middle managers' objectives.

Currently, as far as the consumer empowerment process is concerned, the newly-developed Mental Health Directorate, which incorporates the former QA adviser, has accepted the objectives for information from consumers and to consumers and the involvement of consumers in planning. The newly-developed user group has the charter as one of its tasks and is actively consulting on a final draft before passing it to the statutory agencies for their views. The forum worker has successfully bid for mental health specific grant monies to employ an advocacy worker. There are two research projects which will support the consumerism component. The University of Kent (CAPSC) successfully obtained King's Fund money for a project on user-defined elements of service evaluation in residential projects (Kerruish & Smith, Chapter 7) and the project co-ordinator is liaising closely with the health authority quality worker and the consumer monitoring group. Although the QA money is not available this year, audit money is, and a bid has been made to the regional health authority for audit money for further development of a care planning model which has consumer or advocate involvement and which can be used as an audit tool for individual cases.

Resistance to change

Observing the early interplay between user representatives and senior professionals in the mental health quality review team illustrated that, if one drew up a list of human factors relevant to the change process one might identify fear and anxiety, prejudice, ignorance, rigidity of thinking and lack of motivation for change as being key issues. The irony was that both professionals and user representatives showed these features to an equal degree. In the inner London consortium, if one took a parallel situation within the co-ordination group, the lower prevalence of these issues probably reflected the fact that the professionals involved in the activity had done so voluntarily because of their greater motivation to help bring about the change process. It is fair to say that the change process in the outer London area, which began from within the statutory organization, suffered more constraints related to resistance by groups of individuals. One could list virtually every stakeholder: there was significant sabotaging by senior nurse managers; medical professionals had the highest level of anxiety; the carers involved tended towards the bossy and paternalistic; and initially at least, users were rather institutionalized and passive in their attitude. This all made for greater organizational resistance to the process than in the inner London area, where starting from outside the organization as the process did, the main difficulty was that the process was hostage to the current political culture and initially had relative insecurity in regard to its future. However, as previously illustrated, as the process continued, the inner London project has consolidated substantially by having a clear role which the statutory organizations could utilize. Paradoxically though, the strategic model is itself currently in danger of being a hostage to the wide-ranging change processes which come out of the NHS reforms and which present a real danger to the implementation process by diluting its momentum.

If one compares the environmental factors that are influencing the change process in the two areas, there are five features which differ between the two sites and which have a role in influencing progress. Firstly, the outer London area had low mobility of clients and it seemed that as a result, users were more institutionalized and needed greater support and encouragement to form their own group. In the inner London area, the prevailing culture was an activist one and this did seem partially related to relative economic deprivation. On the other hand, the outer London project had the advantage of NHS development money, whereas the inner London project had to struggle with initial status as a charity to obtain appropriate funds. The political culture in the inner London area, on the other hand, was markedly left-wing. This meant that new projects, particularly consumer oriented ones, would be given preferential support although, as noted above, associated risks included the instability of the local culture which tended to produce a lot of new projects that flourished briefly and then died off. In the outer London area, there was a very stable right-wing political culture which was in principle anti-consumer and paternalist. This was also reflected in the next factor – the stance of the local authority. The local authority had a tradition of low investment in community activities. NHS investment in quality suited the local authority perfectly as it saw no reason for additional funds to be made available from its own resources, whereas in the inner London site, the local authority saw it as natural to support a consumer related project. Finally, as noted above, there was a very high level of sabotage in the outer London area by vested interests, although this reflected the development process of a project from within the organization, rather than necessarily any other aspect of prevailing culture. It is probable that the NHS organization in the inner London area

138

would have been equally likely to produce a host of saboteurs had the inner London project not had support on the boundary of the statutory organizations and interests outside them. Within that context the situation was sufficiently disorganized for the possibility of sabotage to be much less.

Conclusion

An overview of the two projects described above reveals four common issues which are extremely familiar to those involved in change management in general. The first, is the strong influence of the pre-existing culture in facilitating or inhibiting the change process. The second, is the time scale concerned. It is quite clear that the kind of culture change that one attempts in introducing consumerism requires a time scale of five to seven years for significant change to be brought about. This is an important factor to be taken into account when attempting to assess, for development purposes, the likely level of resources required for the achievement of the process. The next important common factor is the influence of the external environment. Throughout the course of the projects so far, there has been prevailing impingement on the processes of changes in the external environment, such as the impact of 'Care in the Community', the NHS reforms, etc. which inevitably interact with any implementation process and need to be accommodated. Finally, both projects share a need for one or two highly motivated individuals with vision and energy to help drive the process onwards. Without this momentum, the change process runs the risk of developing all too slowly or even of being dissipated completely. This final point illustrates the risks inherent in any change process. Even with the most careful and detailed planning, without having the fortune to find the right individuals who will carry the process forward, making change a reality becomes a most uncertain activity.

(1)
(2)
(3)
(4)

[handwritten annotations:]

4 issues common to both projects (tend to change management generally).

(1) strong influence of pre-existing culture.

(2) Time scale of 5-7 yrs for significant cultural change.

(3) Influence of external environment. + need for changes there to be accommodated

(4) Need for 1 or 2 + motivated indivs. to drive on change process + keep momentum going. (NB element of luck in getting right people).

139

17 User feedback and organizational change

Rob Leiper

This is a book about change. Directly creating change in mental health services may not be the only grounds for moving towards greater consumer participation and feedback. There is a moral imperative behind the calls for greater openness and fuller empowerment which gives such expectations an obvious rightness. The hope, nevertheless, is that more respectful and caring relationships can be produced within the services by responding to such demands. These are subtle and far-reaching changes within the culture of service delivery, change at the most general level. For the most part, however, the specific methods proposed for attaining and ensuring the empowerment of service users, whether through feedback or representation, have the character of quality assurance systems. They aim at concrete changes in the practice of specific services and they do so by providing new information – feeding back users' reactions to the services they have received and introducing a fresh perspective through user participation in decision making forums. Unfortunately, amidst the methodological ingenuity, the visionary programmes and the public relations 'hype', too little attention is paid to the simple fact that the goal is to create change and that change is never easy – it takes cunning and commitment. Hannu Vuori (1991) of the World Health Organization recently asked whether it has been shown anywhere that collecting information about the satisfaction of service users improves quality in any field of health care. He concludes from a review of the literature that: 'The honest answer is: we do not know.' This lack of evidence reflects, I suspect, an equal lack of attention in practice to ways of ensuring that positive changes actually do result from efforts to involve service users.

This concluding chapter will attempt to sketch out some of the factors which must be attended to and a few of the conditions which should be created in order to maximize our chances of promoting change through introducing the views of consumers into the decision making of mental health services. There is, of course, substantial literature about organizational development and the management of change to draw upon (Bennis, 1969). This makes it more surprising that so little attention has been paid to thinking through these issues. In the terms of these development methodologies, the specific change strategy adopted in consumer participation might be conceived of as generating and feeding back new information. From this perspective, the basic concepts which might help us understand how to proceed most effectively are organizational change and information feedback rather than the various methods and structures which have been used to obtain consumer views. This suggests a more process oriented view of the practical issues and, while running the danger of being overly abstract, it has the strength of enabling many of the problems of effective implementation to be seen in a more clearly defined light. We are then required by this clarity of thinking to be more specific in asking what kind of information is to be sought, what type of change is aimed for and how this change will be effected.

Nadler (1977) suggests that these three questions represent the major aspects of any organizational development programme based around informational feedback (see Figure 1). They can represent different emphases in the creation of such programmes but in order to have the maximum likelihood of success, all three elements require equal attention. It is important not to become overly fascinated by one facet of the process at the expense of the others. Each aspect is related to the others but they will be considered in turn as a means of analyzing the conditions under which consumer feedback programmes will be most likely to succeed.

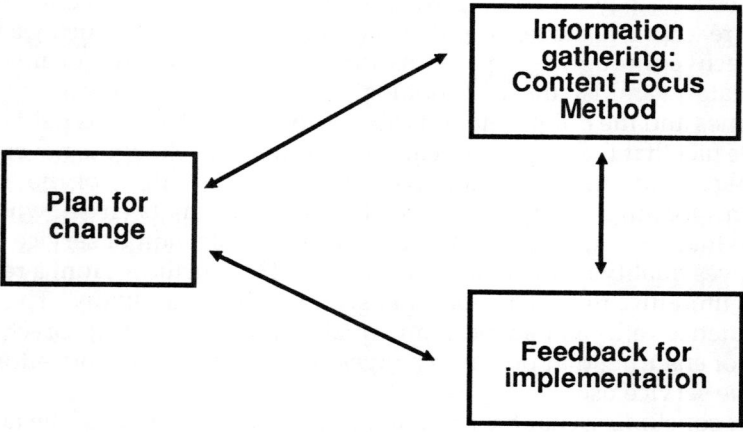

Figure 1 Using Information for Change

142

Since the issue of 'information gathering' – actually obtaining users' views, has been a major focus of this work we shall start there. It must be acknowledged that there is always a temptation not to collect new data, the temptation to think: 'Why bother? We already know what is going to be said.' This is certainly a common reaction amongst staff groups in service settings. Perhaps, however, it can also be a tendency within user participation structures such as patients' councils, users' forums or user representation on planning groups, where there may be a danger of activists assuming that they represent a consensus, or at least the best informed and most progressive viewpoint. Users are individuals and it cannot be assumed that either their needs or their values and viewpoints are all similar. There should always be a sense of obligation on us all to check out these assumptions and be prepared to have them challenged. The need to do this properly then highlights the significance of all those methodological issues regarding how to get accurate information – reliability, validity, representativeness. These issues can easily seem tedious and irrelevant but they apply as much to the process of generating problems and aspirations in a group discussion as they do to a questionnaire in a survey. Yvonne Webb's discussion (Chapter 2) of the difficulties and complexities of these issues points out how relatively little serious attention seems to be paid to them even in the 'survey' tradition. The quality of information is neglected in the face of the pressure just to do something. It is important to think out what information, about what issues and in what form might really be of use to any specific service. From this starting point tough questions can be asked about what methods can be used to obtain it most accurately within the resources of time and energy available.

Perhaps the most important influence on making these decisions should be the purposes of the information. One might describe the reasons for collecting data as being broadly two-fold. In the first place, the intended effect might be to energize and motivate the recipients to take action. Here the main issue is to enable a service to take an issue seriously or to provoke it into reconsidering assumptions. Information should therefore help to establish the need for change in the minds of those who provide the service. However, it is important to consider the direction of the 'energy' created since it is possible to do this in a way which raises anxieties and so increases resistance to change. The aim must be to collect and present data in such a way that the energy will be utilized to identify and solve problems. This points to the second and more obvious function of collecting data, to direct action towards areas in which change is required, enabling learning and goal setting to take place. Here the aim is to guide action towards specific targets which are viewed as a priority and, perhaps subsequently, to monitor how successful the effort has been. Both of these functions are essential and they are a reminder that the process of collecting information is not simply one of assessment (for example measuring aspects of service quality) but should be geared towards use in problem solving: information should be action oriented and lead to further work.

These considerations concerning the response to and use of information have important implications for the type of data that should be collected. Nadler (1977) proposes a list of characteristics which information should have in order to produce maximum impact and likelihood of leading to positive action when it is fed back in the context of any organizational intervention. The desirable qualities are that such information should be:

Relevant	Limited
Understandable	Comparative
Descriptive	Impactive
Verifiable	Unfinalized

Thus some of these qualities amount to the idea that information should 'make sense' to the staff who have to respond to it in terms of their concerns and ways of seeing things. It is desirable for it to be vividly descriptive, by being clear, concrete and specific. Evaluations of the current situation should not be overly judgemental and critical. It is important to avoid both threat and overload. Many of the methods described earlier in this book, and the type of data which they generate, might be appraised in relation to these criteria, since they describe their potential to promote change. One might conclude that many feedback methods produce information which is remote and rather abstract, while some participatory structures must struggle with the trap of being overly critical. Problem oriented action is again the crucial issue in relation to the suggestion that information identify issues within the power of a group to affect (have an impact upon). This is also at the core of the interesting notion that data should merely point the direction for further thought and problem solving rather than being overly complete in themselves.

These considerations lead on to the second major component of information based organizational change programmes: how feedback and implementation opportunities are structured. This element has been a significant focus for those concerned with user participation. It is pointless to undertake information gathering if it is to be fed back without the structures in place for acting upon it. It is, however, quite common. Information should be relevant to the interests and scope of authority for action of the group it is provided to. Preferably there should also be clear systems and resources available through which a response can be made and these should have been considered and put in place beforehand. 'Designs' for both collecting and feeding back information differ considerably and should receive more conscious attention than they typically do. This implies that a working group should be created and authorized to review and act upon information which is collected or an existing group charged with the specific responsibility to do so. These working groups, where they exist, should be created in such a way as to cope productively with the potential conflicts, divisions and resistances to change which are likely to be generated. Thus, groups may consist of staff at only one level in an organization, perhaps with a similar process repeated at different levels (as for example in Jones, Chapter 4); or they may deliberately mix different levels and perspectives within a service (such as described by Kellaher, Chapter 6). It is of course the conviction of many in the users movement that the likelihood of users' views being taken seriously and being acted upon can really only be guaranteed by the inclusion of user representation on the relevant groups. While this may often be the case, there may also be circumstances in which defensiveness will be unfavourably increased by the sense of exposure created by the presence of an 'outsider.' At the same time, a user presence is never a guarantee of effectiveness since as Marion Beeforth points out (Chapter 10) there are all too many ways in which such representation can be undermined and which must be guarded against.

Certainly the membership of such working groups must have been selected so that they share a sense of common problems or else preliminary work must be undertaken to establish some sense of common purpose. Groups should be both motivated to take action on identified problems and clearly empowered to do so. If data is in any way complex or technical it may be important to provide appropriate assistance in interpreting and using it. Group work of this kind is likely to be aided by an agenda and clear structures and decision making procedures rather than their being left entirely open. Finally, it should be recognized that difficulties and conflict are extremely likely, at least over the longer term, and that for any such group to be effective and sustained it may well benefit from some form of facilitation with its own process (such as proposed by Pilling through the role of 'quality reviewer', Chapter 5).

All of these considerations with respect to the form of information gathering and to the structures for feeding back and acting on it emphasize that there are numerous options and choices to be made in designing an effective consumer feedback programme. Attention to these is crucial since the decisions made affect the likelihood of promoting constructive change in a service. They relate to the third facet of the overall programme: creating a plan for change. However, one has the impression that very often little real planning takes place and that such design decisions are not made consciously but by default.

Planning for change involves defining to some degree what you hope will be your destination and how you intend to get there. This thought-through relationship between the aims of a programme and the steps by which these will be reached is often striking by its absence. The difficulties of effecting organizational change are well known and yet change in response to feedback is often taken for granted. This seems particularly true of those models which depend on consumer satisfaction surveys, where there is a largely untested assumption that appropriate and effective action will result from simply collecting information. It may be helpful to keep in mind a simple schematic overview of the elements of a strategic approach to planned change which can act as a guide to these issues in designing user involvement programmes. Plant (1987) proposes the following 'steps to change':

- establish the need for change;
- create a (shared) vision of change;
- assess the readiness for change;
- create a strategy for change designed to: build influence, and overcome resistance.

It is perhaps the greatest achievement of the users movement that, together with professional critics of the system, it has been able to establish and reinforce in the minds of many that change is needed within mental health services. This has been done by a variety of means including publicizing the work of empirical researchers and the findings of a series of hospital scandal investigations, publicizing many moving accounts of personal experience and backing all this by vigorous political campaigning. This change in perception has been the result of a long and arduous effort by many concerned users and their carers, by professionals and researchers, lobbyists and regulatory authorities alike. The users movement has also articulated the vision of change: one centred around respectful treatment, due regard for civil rights, access to resources, partnership and involvement. However, it has be recognized that there is no clear consensus around this vision or what it should mean in practice. There are differences of emphasis within the users movement, differences between users and their carers and differences both from and amongst the perspectives of various professionals and service managers. A shared consensus cannot be created by simply assuming or asserting it exists. It seems likely that a vision of a better service will need to be negotiated and renegotiated repeatedly within each service setting as well as within the wider community. Conflicts and differences which are simply ignored or suppressed will return to sabotage well-intended changes. As Richard Grover points out (in Chapter 8), it is tempting to use power to take a direct route to enforce change since the process of mediating and negotiating differences can be slow and painful but the easy road is not necessarily the one which leads to sustainable development.

In order to know how to move forward it is important to be clear-sighted about where a service is currently situated. There can be no universally applicable strategy for turning a service into one which is more responsive to its users. Sadly, we always have to start each journey from where we are now! We must ask what this service is realistically capable of doing as its first steps. Yet assessing this is seldom easy and may not be particularly encouraging. It will certainly involve complex and contradictory elements. While service commissioners point out that the new contracting arrangements provide important new mechanisms for influencing the pattern of service provision (Raftery and Barker, Chapters 12 and 13), the 'turbulence' in the organizational environment created by the sweeping changes in management structures and through the competitive, cash-regulated environment of the internal market also has significant detrimental effects to enabling creative change. David Somekh (Chapter 16) has illustrated how such internal reorganization over-

Driving Forces →	Resisting Forces ←
Need to obtain/threat of losing contracts and accreditation leading to:	Not knowing there is a problem
	Not knowing what problem is
demands from boards and managers for performance goals	Lack of resources
	Poor service quality
Image/reputation with community groups, with peer groups (= cultural change)	Low sense of rewards for change
	Threat to current rewards (including power/status)
Complaints	Low morale & high uncertainty
Desire of staff to provide good service	Exposure to emotional threats
Moral concern	

Figure 2 Force Field Analysis

takes and disrupts even carefully planned change programmes. One simple way of assessing the readiness of an organization for change and gaining a clearer picture of an inevitably complex situation is to undertake a force field analysis. While this should certainly be done for each individual service a sketch of the factors which bear generally on many services at this time is presented in Figure 2. This represents those forces positively supporting and pressing for change and the opposing factors which are likely to resist or inhibit development. Building influence involves identifying developmental forces within the organizational environment and allying with those elements likely to be supportive of them.

This brief portrait of competing forces within an organizational environment suggests the considerable difficulty lying in the path of creating more responsive and respectful services. Many of the tensions and conflicts which can create resistance are intrinsic to the nature of mental health services. They may be divided into 'external' and 'internal' sources of conflict. The external conflicts represent differences in the interests of different groups and to some extent these underlie the differences in perspective which prevent any easy achievement of consensus. These issues concern (or are, at least felt to concern) 'who wins' and 'who loses' from change, whose interests are seen as central and who has the most power to define the agenda and control resources. It is all too easy to overlook the degree to which the exercise of power is crucial in these 'negotiations' about a dominant definition of social 'reality'. The interests of sufferers and carers are not necessarily identical. The interests of the wider society are influential both in terms of the wish to limit funding and the demand on services to exercise a function of social control. Professionals too have legitimate sectional interests to be rewarded and validated in their roles and provided with the support and authority to perform them. Any definition of a service is the outcome therefore of a 'political' process. In particular, there are currently intense and sometimes destructive battles for influence and control being waged between professionals and a new class of managers within services: consumers are in some danger of being 'cannon fodder' in this war. There are also struggles between users and carers (both 'consumers') to define services, giving precedence to their own perspective but again sometimes exploited in the pursuit of inter-professional rivalries. It is the achievement of the users movement to have greatly increased the visibility and political influence of the recipients of mental health services within the public sphere. This goes far beyond personal empowerment but it falls and, I believe, must fall short of a totally 'consumer oriented' (still less consumer controlled) mental health system. That the mental health services can function entirely in the self-defined interests of those who directly receive them is a myth, a myth which may be currently helpful

148

in many circumstances, but one which can become a piece of politically motivated mystification which should be resisted. The conflicts of interest are real, will remain and are better discussed than ignored.

It seems particularly important to face these external difficulties because they interact with and are further fuelled by the internal, 'felt' conflicts and resistances which are inevitably stirred up in all concerned with the experience of mental illness and emotional distress. In particular, these include not only feelings of fear, outrage and grief but also of powerlessness, which can affect everyone: not only sufferers who feel their lives invaded by an alien experience; but also carers, professionals and managers who feel unable to help enough. The nature of the distress thus caused can create intense emotional and interpersonal pressures which are likely to be dealt with defensively and can often be enacted through destructive institutional practices and chronic splits between different groups within the service. These defensive processes will often be at the root of neglectful or abusive care practices and of the reluctance to change them. The users of mental health services have suffered for many years by being at the receiving end of such processes. There continues to be a temptation to deal with this often fraught situation by getting into further fights, setting up good guys and bad guys and so simplifying a confusingly complicated and difficult situation. Overly simple calls for 'empowerment' can be a denial of how desperate people are feeling. Real respect for the voice of users can only be achieved through the struggle for empathic understanding, mutual respect and the toleration of differing points of view.

To this extent, a tone of excessive certainty and zealous conviction may be unhelpful and an effort to impose solutions will contain the seeds of its own failure. It is too easy to assume that certain means (for example, user representation) are identical to the ends they are intended to achieve; or that simply instituting certain procedures (for example, consumer feedback arrangements) will inevitably and naturally lead to those ends. Clarity of expectations and the creation of appropriate demands and constraints (for example, in service contracts) are, of course, important and not the same as imposing a point of view. However, the more important aspects of the process of commissioning a more consumer oriented service may be the careful thought, the negotiation and the conscious planning which should go into agreeing and implementing a strategy for change. It is such a considered attitude towards the process of influencing interested parties within a service which often seems striking by its absence. This seems to represent a failure of true respect, a failure to take things seriously enough.

Such a strategic approach would endeavour not merely to increase the penalties for failing to achieve targets concerned with user responsiveness but would attempt to encourage and reward positive developments rather than simply pressurize services. Moreover, it would pay attention not only to attempting to increase forces which promote change but to actively reducing the potential resistances. If this is not done the attempt to push for change can create an equal and opposite reaction against it. This can be represented by a superficial compliance with the letter of these demands, while the spirit becomes simply one of public relations. Positive concern for others and the natural wish to feel effective in one's work are indispensable allies within staff groups which can help to create real, internalized – rather than compliant – change. Reducing resistance within service-providing organizations is likely to involve increasing the felt security of the people within them. In this way it may be more possible to reduce the atmosphere of defensiveness and to enable organizational boundaries to become more permeable to new information and points of view. Feedback and possible change need not then be experienced simply as a threat. Without this atmosphere quality assurance systems, consumer feedback and user participation structures will be undertaken tokenistically and function merely as a new form of institutional defence mechanism.

People use mental health services because they go through times in their life when they are in extremes of desperation. They are surely not primarily interested in ideologies and structures but in services and relationships, perhaps most significantly in the respectful availability of those individuals charged with providing care. It is 'feedback' and 'empowerment' at this level which more than anything else would meet these demands. To provide this, service organizations must be capable of transforming themselves into the holders and nurturers of a culture which enables such relationships. If the aim is to create a climate in which services become more open and responsive to their users at all levels, then the means of achieving it must be to create circumstances within organizations in which differences are tolerated, dialogue encouraged and an openness to learning valued above all else. This means knowing that we don't know all the answers. It means listening and thinking carefully and seriously about what we hear and what we do.

Bibliography

Abrahamson, D. and Brenner, D., (1982), 'Do Long-stay Psychiatric Patients Want to Leave Hospital?', *Health Trends*, 14, 95 – 97.

Abrahamson, D., Swatton, J. and Wills, W., (1989), 'Do long-stay Psychiatric Patients Want to Leave Hospital?', *Health Trends*, 21, 17 – 19

Alcock, J. and Brown, H., (1989), *New Lifestyles*, Pavilion Publishing, Brighton.

Anderson, J., (1989), 'Patient Power in Mental Health', *British Medical Journal*, 299, 1477 – 1488.

Armstrong, D., (1991), 'What Do Patients Want?', *British Medical Journal*, 303, 261 – 262.

Baggott, R., (1988), 'Pressure Group Politics in Britain: Change and Decline?' *Talking Politics*, 1, 25 – 29.

Barker, I. and Peck, E., (1988), 'Power in Strange Places: User Empowerment in Mental Health Services', *Good Practices in Mental Health*, GPMH, London.

Beeforth, M., Conlan, E., Hoser, B. and Sayce, L., (1990), *Whose Service Is It Anyway? Users' Views on Co-ordinating Care.*, RDP, London.

Bender, M. P. and Pilling, S., (1985), 'A Study of Variables Associated with Under-Attendance at a Psychiatric Day Hospital', *Psychological Medicine*, 15, 395 – 402.

Bennis, N. G., (1969), *Organization Development: its Nature, Origins and Prospects*, Addison-Wesley, Reading, Ma.

Bhugra, D., (1989), 'Attitudes Towards Mental Illness. A Review of the Literature', *Acta Psychiatrica Scandinavica*, 80, 1 – 12.

Biggs, S., (1990), 'Consumers, Case Management and Inspection', *Critical Social Policy*, 30, 23 – 28.

Brown, P., (1981), 'The Mental Patients' Rights Movement and Mental Health Institutional Change', *International Journal of Health Services*, 11, 523 – 540.

Buckland, I., (1988), 'Power Through Partnership: an Account of the Contact Group in Chesterfield', In Barker, I. and Peck, E. (eds) *Power in Strange Places: User Empowerment in Mental Health Services,* GPMH, London.

Camden Mental Health Consortium, (1986), *Mental Health Priorities in Camden as We See Them: The Consumer Viewpoint,* CMHC, London.

Carr, J., Stingsley, R. and Raftery, J., (1990), 'Preferential Insights', *Health Service Journal,* Nov. 22, 1732 – 1733.

Chamberlin, J., (1988), *On Our Own,* MIND, London.

Clifford, P. and Webb, Y., (1991), *The Face Project.* For Details contact Paul Clifford, Quality Development Unit, 58, Ling's Coppice, Croxted Road, London SE21 8SX.

Clifford, P., Leiper, R., Lavender, A. and Pilling, S., (1989), *The QUARTZ System: Assuring Quality in Mental Health Settings,* RDP/Free Associations, London.

Corrigan, P. W., (1990), 'Consumer Satisfaction with Institutional and Community Care', *Community Health Journal,* 26, 151 – 165.

Corrigan, P. W., Liberman, R. P. and Engel, J. D., (1990), 'From Non-compliance to Collaboration in the Treatment of Schizophrenia', *Hospital and Community Psychiatry,* 41, 1203 – 1211.

Davidson, L., (1989), *Taking the Steam out of the Team,* Pavilion Publishing, Brighton.

Dyer, L., (1990), *The Right to Vote,* North West MIND.

East Anglia RHA/Office of Public Management, (1990), *Contracting for Health Outcomes,* East Anglia RHA, Cambridge.

Elbeck, M. and Fecteau, G., (1990), 'Improving the Validity of Measures of Patient Satisfaction with Psychiatric Care and Treatment', *Hospital and Community Psychiatry,* 41, 998 – 1001.

Fenton, F. R., Tessier, L. and Struering, E. L., (1979), 'A Comparative Trial of Home and Hospital Psychiatric Care. One Year Follow-up', *Archives Of General Psychiatry,* 36, 1073 – 1079.

Finlay-Jones, R., (1983), 'The Practice of Psychiatry in the Community', *Australian and New Zealand Journal of Psychiatry,* 17, 107 – 108.

Fitzpatrick, R., (1991), 'Audit in Person: Surveys of Patient Satisfaction: II – Designing a Questionnaire and Conducting a Survey', *British Medical Journal,* 302, 1129 – 1132.

Goldberg, D. and Huxley, P., (1980), *Mental Illness in the Community. The Pathway to Psychiatric Care,* Tavistock, London

Gordon, D., Alexander, A. and Dietzan, J., (1979), 'The Psychiatric Patient: a Voice to be Heard', *British Journal of Psychiatry,* 135, 115 – 121.

GPMH and Camden Mental Health Consortium, (1989), *Treated Well? – A Code of Practice for Psychiatric Hospitals,* GPMH and CMHC, London.

Gregoire, P. A., (1990), 'The Phenomenology of Psychiatric Hospitalization: the Patient's Experience and Expectations', *Acta Psychiatrica Scandinavica,* 82, 210 – 212.

Hansson, L., (1989), 'Patient Satisfaction With In-hospital Psychiatric Care',

European Archives of Psychiatric and Neurological Sciences, 239, 93 – 100.

HMSO, (1992), *Ashworth Report: Report of Inquiry into Complaints About Ashworth Hospital,* London.

HMSO, (1989b), *Caring for People,* London.

HMSO, (1991), *Health of the Nation* – Green Paper, London.

HMSO, (1992), *Health of the Nation* – White Paper, London.

HMSO, (1991), *Patients' Charter,* London.

HMSO, (1988), *Residential Care: a Positive Choice, Report of the Independent Review of Residential Care,* Chaired by Gillian Wagner.

HMSO, (1989a), *Working for Patients,* London.

Hill, R. and Leiper, R., (1992), *Evaluating Quality Assurance: a Report of the Research Evaluation of the QUARTZ System,* RDP, London.

Holcomb, W. R,, Adams, N. A., Ponder, H. M., Reitz, R., (1989), 'The Development and Construction of a Consumer Satisfaction Questionnaire for Psychiatric In-patients', *Evaluation and Program Planning,* 12, 189 – 194.

Holloway, F. (1991), 'Case Management for the Mentally Ill : Looking at the Evidence', *International Journal of Social Psychiatry,* 37, 1, 2 – 13.

Holloway, F., (1989), 'Psychiatric Day Care: The Users' Perspective', *International Journal of Social Psychiatry,* 35, 252 – 264.

Hoult, J., Reynolds, I., Charbounneau-Powis, M., Weekes, P. and Briggs, J., (1983), 'Psychiatric Hospital Versus Community Treatment: Results of a Randomised Trial', *Australian and New Zealand Journal of Psychiatry,* 17, 160 – 167.

Huxley, P., (1980), *User Satisfaction Survey,* (UnPub).

Huxley, P. and Mohamad, H., (1991), *Global Satisfaction Measure (GMS – 1),* Mental Health Social Work Research Unit, Manchester University.

Hyde-Price, C., (1986), *Our User's Voice – the Effect of Patient Opinion Surveys on the Management of Health Service,* Unpublished report for the National Management Training Scheme.

Illich, I., (1977), *Limits to Medicine: Medical Nemesis: the Expropriation of Health,* Pelican (Penguin) Books, Harmondsworth.

International Hospital Federation, (1988), *And What Would They Know About It: the Issues, Options and Implications of Seeking the Patient's Point of View,* International Hospital Federation, London.

Jones, L., Leneman, L. and Maclean, U., (1987), *Consumer Feedback for the NHS. A Literature Review,* King's Fund, London.

Kay, A. and Legg, C., (1986), *Discharged to the Community,* Housing Research Group, The City University, London.

Kelman, H. R., (1976), 'Evaluation of Health Care Quality by Consumers', *International Journal of Health Services,* 6, 431 – 442.

Kelman, H. R., (1967), 'Human Use of Human Subjects: the Problem of Deception in Social Psychological Experiments', *Psychological Bulletin,* 1 – 14. Reprinted in Bynner, J. and Stribley, K. (Eds.), (1979), *Social*

Research; Principles and Procedures, Lygman and Open University Press.

Kingsley, S. and Towell, D., (1988), 'Planning for High-quality Local Services', In A. Lavender and F. Holloway (eds) *Community Care in Practice,* Wiley, Chichester.

Lambeth MIND, (1988), *Thoughts of Home: The Views of Your Consumers,* MIND, London.

Lebow, J. L., (1974), 'Consumer Assessments of the Quality of Medical Care', *Medical Care,* 12, 328 – 337.

Lebow, J., (1982), 'Consumer Satisfaction With Mental Health Treatment', *Psychological Bulletin,* 91, 244 – 259.

Lee, H. S., (1979), 'Patients' Comments on Psychiatric In-patient Treatment Experiences: Patient – Therapist Relationships and Their Implications for Treatment Outcome', *Psychiatric Quarterly,* 51, 39.

Lehman, A. F., Reed, S. K. and Possiennte, S. M., (1982a), 'Priorities for Long-term Care: Comments from Board and Care Residents', *Psychiatric Quarterly,* 54, 181 – 189.

Lehman, A. F., Ward, N., Linn, L. S., (1982b), 'Chronic Mental Patients: the Quality of Life Issue', *American Journal of Psychiatry,* 139, 1271 – 1276.

Lehman, A. F., (1983), 'The Well-being of Chronic Mental Patients', *Archives of General Psychiatry,* 40, 369 – 373.

Leiper, R., Pilling, S. Lavender, A. and Clifford, P., (1992a), *Implementing a Quality Review System,* Pavilion Publishing, Brighton.

Leiper, R., Lavender, A., Pilling, S. and Clifford, P., (1992b), *The QUARTZ Schedules,* Pavilion Publishing, Brighton.

Leiper, R., Pilling, S. and Lavender, A., (1992c), *Using the QUARTZ Schedules,* Pavilion Publishing, Brighton.

Leitman, R., Morrison, I. and Donelan, K., (1990), 'Satisfaction With Health Systems in Ten Nations', *Health Affairs,* 9, 185 – 192.

Lieberman, P. B. and Strauss, J. S., (1986), 'Psychiatric Hospitalization: What are its Effects?', *American Journal of Psychiatry,* 143, 1557 – 1562.

Locker, D. and Dunt, D., (1978), 'Theoretical and Methodological Issues in Sociological Studies of Consumer Satisfaction With Medical Care', *Social Science and Medicine,* 12, 283 – 292.

Lorefice, L. S. and Borus, J. F., (1984), 'Consumer Evaluation of a Community Mental Health Service II: Perceptions of Clinical Care', *American Journal of Psychiatry,* 141, 1449 – 1452.

MacCarthy, B., Benson, J. and Brewin, C. R., (1986), 'Task Motivation and Problem Appraisal in Long-Term Psychiatric Patients', *Psychological Medicine,* 16, 431 – 438.

MacCarthy, B., (1988), 'The Role of Relatives', In A. Lavender and F. Holloway (eds) *Community Care in Practice,* Wiley, Chichester.

Macdonald, L., Sibbald, B., and Hoare, C., (1988),'Measuring Patient Satisfaction With Life in a Long-stay Psychiatric Hospital', *The International Journal of Social Psychiatry,* 34, 292 – 304.

McIver, S., (1991), *Obtaining the Views of Users of Mental Health Services,* King's Fund Centre, London.

McKnight, J., (1977), 'Professionalised Service and Disabling Help', in *Disabling Professions,* Marion Boyars, London.

Mayer, J. E. and Rosenblatt, A., (1974), 'Clash in Perspective Between Mental Patients and Staff', *American Journal of Orthopsychiatry,* 44, 4 – 32.

MIND and the Roehampton Institute, (1990), *People First,* MIND, London

MIND, (1992), *Stress on Women Campaign Pack,* MIND, London.

Mosher, L., Burti, L., (1989), *Community Mental Health : Principles and Practice,* Norton, New York.

Nader, R., (1972), *Unsafe at Any Speed,* Grossman, New York.

Nadler, D., (1977), *Feedback and Organisation Development: Using Data Based Methods,* Addison-Wesley, Reading, Ma.

O'Donnell, O., Maynard, A. and Wright, K., (1988), *The Economic Evaluation of Mental Health Care: a Review,* York Centre for Health Economics, York.

Oppenheim, A. N., (1966), *Questionnaire Design and Attitude Measurement,* Heinemann Books on Sociology, UK.

Pampling, D., (1991), 'The New NHS', *British Medical Journal,* 302, 737 – 738.

Pickard, L., Proudfoot, R., Woolfson, P., Clifford, P., Holloway, F., and Lindesay, J., (1992), *Evaluating the Closure of Cane Hill Hospital, Mental Health Services in the Community, New Services in the Context of Hospital Closure,* RDP, London.

Piersma, H. L., (1986), 'Patient Comments Concerning Psychiatric Hospitalization', *Psychiatric Quarterly,* 58, 32 – 41.

Pilgrim, D. and Rogers, A., (1990), 'User-Friendly Research', *Openmind,* 45, 4 – 5.

Plant, R., (1987), *Managing Change and Making it Stick,* Fontana, London.

Potter, J., (1988), 'Consumerism in the Public Sector: How Well Does the Coat Fit?', *Public Administration,* 66, 149 – 164.

Pugh, R., (1990), *Obtaining the Consumer's View on Psychiatric Services: a Client-Centred Approach – A Particular Challenge for Psychiatry,* Unpublished paper. St Luke's Woodside Hospital, Muswell Hill, London, N10 3HU.

Raftery, J. and Zarb, G., (1990), 'Satisfaction guaranteed?', *Health Service Journal,* Nov. 15, 1692 – 1693.

Ramon, S., (1991), *Action Research,* Paper presented at the seminar on Action Research of the Mental Health Research Network, December 16th, at RDP.

Ramon, S., (1991), personal communication.

Ramon, S., (1985), *Psychiatry in Britain : Meaning and Policy,* Croom Helm, London.

Raphael, W., (1972), *Psychiatric Hospitals Viewed by their Patients*, King Edward's Hospital Fund for London, London.

Romme, M. A. J. and Escher, A. D. M. A. C., (1989), 'Hearing Voices', *Schizophrenia Bulletin*, 15, 209 – 216.

Royal College of Psychiatrists, (1989), 'Patient Advocacy Report for Public Policy Committee', *Psychiatric Bulletin*, 13, 715 – 716.

Ryan, P., (1991), *Dilemmas in Past and Present Action Research in Mental Health*. Paper presented at the above seminar, December 16th.

Sang, R. and O'Brien, J., (1984), 'Advocacy: The UK and American Experience', *King's Fund Project Paper 51*, King's Fund Centre, London.

Scull, A., (1978), *Decarceration*, Prentice Hall, Englewood Ciff, New Jersey.

Scull, A., (1984), *Decarceration: Community Treatment and the Deviant: a Radical View*, Polity Press, Cambridge.

Scull, A. T., (1979), *Museums of Madness*, Penguin, Harmondsworth.

Shepherd, D., (1990), 'Following the Code', *Open Mind*, June/July 1990, 9.

Shields, P. J., Morrison, P. and Hart, D., (1988), 'Consumer Satisfaction on a Psychiatric Ward', *Journal of Advanced Nursing*, 13, 396 – 400.

Shields, P., (1985), 'The Consumer's View of Psychiatry', *Hospital and Health Services Review*, 81, 117 – 119.

Simpson, M., Buckman, R., Stewart, M., Maguire, P., Lipkin, M., Novack, D., Till, J., (1991), 'Doctor-Patient Communication – the Toronto consensus statement', *British Medical Journal*, 303, 1385 – 1387.

Slater, V., Linn, M. W. and Harris, R., (1982), 'A Satisfaction With Mental Health Care Scale', *Comprehensive Psychiatry*, 23, 68 – 74.

South East MIND, (1990), *Users Participation Pack*, MIND Publications, London.

Stacey, M., (1976), 'The Health Service Consumer: a Sociological Misconception', *Sociological Review*, 22, 194 – 200.

Stein, L. I. and Test, M. A., (1980), *Alternatives to Mental Hospital Treatment*, Plenium Press, New York.

Survivors Speak Out, (1990), *Self Advocacy Pack*, King's Fund, London.

Tolkington, P., (1991), *Black Health : A Political Issue*, Catholic Association for Radical Justice/Liverpool Institute of Higher Education.

Vuori, H., (1991), 'Patient Satisfaction – Does it Matter?', *Quality Assurance in Health Care*, 3(3), 183 – 189.

Waismann, L. C., and Rowland, L. A., (1989), 'Ranking of Needs: A New Method of Assessment for Use With Chronic Psychiatric Patients', *Acta Psychiatrica Scandinavica*.

Ware, J., Davies-Avery, A., Stewart, A., (1978), 'The Measurement and Meaning of Patient Satisfaction', *Health and Medical Care Services Review*, 1, 2 – 14.

Weinstein, R., (1981), 'Attitudes Toward Psychiatric Treatment Among Hospitalized Patients: a Review of Quantitative Research', *Social*

Science and Medicine, 15E, 301 – 314.

Wertheimer, A., (1989), *Building Better Futures; Report of a National SEARCH Conference on the Prospects for Community Mental Health Care*, MIND, London.

Wickings, I., (1989), 'Proof of the Pudding', *Health Service Journal*, 99, 170 – 171.

Whittaker, C., (1986), 'Integrating Formal and Informal Social Care : A Conceptual Framework', *British Journal of Social Work*, Supplement, 16, 41 – 62.

Wilhelm, R., (1951), translation, *I Ching*, Routledge & Kegan Paul, London.

Willcocks, D., Peace, S., and Kellaher, L., (1987), *Private Lives in Public Places: A Research-based Critique of Residential Life in Local Authority Old People's Homes*, Tavistock, London.

Wollstonecraft, M., (1792), *A Vindication Of The Rights Of Woman*, London.

A copy of the QUARTZ schedules and associated manuals can be obtained from

Pavilion Publishing
42 Lansdowne Place
Hove
BN3 IHH

Tel   (0273) 821650
Price   £95.00 (+VAT).

Enquiries concerning the development and training in use of the QUARTZ system should be addressed to

RDP
134/138 Borough High St
London
SE1 1LB

Tel   (071) 403 8790

A list of all MIND's polices, leaflets and other publications is available from:

MIND
Policy Department
22 Harley St
London
W1N 2ED